T0228997

Palliative Therapy in Otolaryngology - Head and Neck Surgery

Guest Editors

KENNETH M. GRUNDFAST, MD, FACS
GEOFFREY P. DUNN, MD, FACS

OTOLARYNGOLOGIC CLINICS OF NORTH AMERICA

www.oto.theclinics.com

February 2009 • Volume 42 • Number 1

SAUNDERS an imprint of ELSEVIER, Inc.

W.B. SAUNDERS COMPANY

A Division of Elsevier Inc.

1600 John F. Kennedy Boulevard ● Suite 1800 ● Philadelphia, Pennsylvania 19103-2899

http://www.theclinics.com

OTOLARYNGOLOGIC CLINICS OF NORTH AMERICA Volume 42, Number 1
February 2009 ISSN 0030-6665, ISBN-13: 978-1-4377-0516-4, ISBN-10: 1-4377-0516-2

Editor: Joanne Husovski
Developmental Editor: Donald Mumford

Otolaryngologic Clinics of North America (ISSN 0030–6665) is published bimonthly by Elsevier Inc., 360 Park Avenue South, New York, NY 10010-1710. Months of issue are February, April, June, August, October, and December. Business and Editorial Offices: 1600 John F. Kennedy Blvd., Suite 1800, Philadelphia, PA 19103-2899. Customer Service Office: 6277 Sea Harbor Drive, Orlando, FL 32887-4800. Periodicals postage paid at New York, NY and additional mailing offices. Subscription price is $264.00 per year (US individuals), $488.00 per year (US institutions), $129.00 per year (US student/resident), $347.00 per year (Canadian individuals), $613.00 per year (Canadian institutions), $390.00 per year (international individuals), $613.00 per year (international institutions), $199.00 per year (international & Canadian student/resident). Foreign air speed delivery is included in all *Clinics'* subscription prices. All prices are subject to change without notice. **POSTMASTER:** Send address changes to *Otolaryngologic Clinics of North America*, Elsevier Periodicals Customer Service, 11830 Westline Industrial Drive, St. Louis, MO 63146. **Customer Service: 1-800-654-2452 (US). From outside the United States, call 1-314-453-7041. Fax: 1-314-453-5170. E-mail: JournalsCustomerService-usa@elsevier.com (for print support) and journalsonlinesupport-usa@elsevier.com (for online support).**

Reprints. For copies of 100 or more of articles in this publication, please contact the Commercial Reprints Department, Elsevier Inc., 360 Park Avenue South, New York, NY 10010-1710. Tel.: 212-633-3812; Fax: 212-462-1935; E-mail: reprints@elsevier.com.

Otolaryngologic Clinics of North America is also published in Spanish by McGraw-Hill Interamericana Editores S.A., P.O. Box 5-237, 06500 Mexico D.F., Mexico.

Otolaryngologic Clinics of North America is covered in *MEDLINE/PubMed (Index Medicus)*, *Current Contents/ Clinical Medicine*, *Excerpta Medica*, *BIOSIS*, *Science Citation Index*, and *ISI/BIOMED*.

Printed and bound in the United Kingdom

Transferred to Digital Print 2011

Contributors

GUEST EDITORS

KENNETH M. GRUNDFAST, MD, FACS
Professor and Chairman, Department Otolaryngology-Head and Neck Surgery, Boston University School of Medicine and the Boston Medical Center, Boston, Massachusetts

GEOFFREY P. DUNN, MD, FACS
Department of Surgery and Palliative Care Consultation Service, Hamot Medical Center, Erie, Pennsylvania

AUTHORS

TERESA CHAN, MD
Department of Otolaryngology—Head and Neck Surgery, Boston University School of Medicine, Boston, Massachusetts

SETH M. COHEN, MD, MPH
Division of Otolaryngology—Head and Neck Surgery, Duke University, Durham, North Carolina

L. CLARKE COX, PhD
Chief of Audiology, Boston Medical Center; Associate Professor, Department of Otolaryngology, Boston University School of Medicine, Boston, Massachusetts

CRAIG DERKAY, MD
Department of Otolaryngology—Head and Neck Surgery, and Department of Pediatrics, Eastern Virginia Medical School, Norfolk, Virginia

ANAND K. DEVAIAH, MD, FACS
Assistant Professor, Department of Otolaryngology—Head and Neck Surgery, and Department of Neurological Surgery, Boston University School of Medicine, Boston, Massachusetts

GEOFFREY P. DUNN, MD, FACS
Department of Surgery and Palliative Care Consultation Service, Hamot Medical Center, Erie, Pennsylvania

ALPHI ELACKATTU, MD
Department of Otolaryngology—Head and Neck Surgery, Boston University Medical Center, Boston, Massachusetts

BARBARA GOLDSTEIN, PhD
Clinical Assistant Professor of Otolaryngology, State University of New York, Downstate, Brooklyn; Director of Audiology, Martha Entenmann Tinnitus Research Center, Inc., Forest Hills, New York

GREGORY GRILLONE, MD, FACS
Associate Professor and Vice Chairman, Department of Otolaryngology, Boston University Medical Center, Boston, Massachusetts

KENNETH M. GRUNDFAST, MD, FACS
Professor and Chairman, Department Otolaryngology—Head and Neck Surgery, Boston University School of Medicine and the Boston Medical Center, Boston, Massachusetts

COURTNEY D. HALL, PhD, PT
Research Health Scientist, Atlanta VAMC, Rehabilitation Research and Development Center, Decatur; Assistant Professor, Department of Rehabilitation Medicine, Emory University, Atlanta, Georgia

SCHARUKH JALISI, MD
Director, Division of Head and Neck Surgical Oncology and Skullbase Surgery; Assistant Professor, Department of Otolaryngology—Head and Neck Surgery, Department of Neurosurgery, Boston University Medical Center, Boston, Massachusetts

KAALAN JOHNSON, MD
Department of Otolaryngology—Head and Neck Surgery, Eastern Virginia Medical School, Norfolk, Virginia

ALEXA T. KOZAK, AuD
Associate Clinical Director, Division of Audiology, Boston University School of Medicine and the Boston Medical Center, Boston, Massachusetts

DENIS LAFRENIERE, MD, FACS
Professor of Surgery and Chief, Division of Otolaryngology, Department of Surgery, University of Connecticut Health Center, Farmington, Connecticut

SUSAN E. LANGMORE, PhD
Professor, Department of Otolaryngology—Head and Neck Surgery, Boston University Medical Center, Boston, Massachusetts

ELIZABETH J. MAHONEY, MD
Assistant Professor, Department of Otolaryngology—Head and Neck Surgery, Boston University School of Medicine, Boston, Massachusetts

NORMAN MANN, MD
Assistant Professor, Department of Medicine; Medical Director, Taste and Smell Clinic, University of Connecticut Health Center, Farmington, Connecticut

ABDEL-KADER MEHIO, MD
Assistant Professor, Department of Anesthesiology, Boston University Medical Center, Boston, Massachusetts

RALPH METSON, MD
Clinical Professor, Department of Otology and Laryngology, Harvard Medical School, Boston, Massachusetts

JAMES L. NETTERVILLE, MD
Director Head and Neck Surgical Oncology; Professor, Department of Otolaryngology—Head and Neck Surgery, Vanderbilt University Medical Center, Nashville, Tennessee

J. PIETER NOORDZIJ, MD
Department of Otolaryngology—Head and Neck Surgery, Boston University Medical Center, Boston, Massachusetts

MICHAEL J. RUCKENSTEIN, MD, MSc, FACS, FRCSC
Professor, Vice-Chairman, Department of Otorhinolaryngology—Head and Neck Surgery, University of Pennsylvania Health System, Philadelphia, Pennsylvania

SWAPNEEL K. SHAH, MD
Resident, Department of Anesthesiology, Boston University Medical Center, Boston, Massachusetts

ABRAHAM SHULMAN, MD, FACS
Professor Emeritus of Clinical Otolaryngology, State University of New York, Downstate, Brooklyn; Director of Otology/Neurotology, Martha Entenmann Tinnitus Research Center, Inc., Forest Hills, New York

JEFFREY P. STAAB, MD, MS
Associate Professor, Departments of Psychiatry, Otorhinolaryngology—Head and Neck Surgery, and Family Medicine and Community Health, University of Pennsylvania Health System, Philadelphia, Pennsylvania

MICHAEL WALSH, MA
Department of Otolaryngology—Head and Neck Surgery, Boston University Medical Center, Boston, Massachusetts

Contents

> The concept of palliation is as old as surgery itself, perhaps so old that it has been taken for granted rather than conceptualized as a primary framework for surgical care. The experience and success of the hospice movement in the United States and abroad was followed by the extension of its basic concepts to the much larger population of patients with advanced, but not necessarily terminal, illness. This collective experience has provided the necessary background and stimulus for developing a specific set of principles and competencies applicable to surgical palliative care. Surgical palliative care is the treatment of suffering and the promotion of quality of life for seriously or terminally ill patients under surgical care.

> This article integrates the highlights of the authors' clinical experiences derived from existing protocols for tinnitus diagnosis and treatment with the evolving discipline of palliation medicine. Specifically, it demonstrates how the inclusion of principles of palliation medicine contributes to the efficacy of treatment.

> Most otolaryngologists encounter patients with chronic rhinosinusitis who, despite conventional medical and surgical therapy, fail to show significant

symptomatic improvement. Many paradigms have been proposed to explain the mechanisms responsible for refractory disease in these patients, including superantigen activation, biofilm formation, and eosinophil activation triggered by fungal elements. Although the precise underlying etiology of this clinical scenario remains unclear, the resultant pathophysiologic events share a final common pathway marked by inflammatory changes of the sinonasal mucosa. This article reviews the proposed hypotheses as to why some patients with chronic sinusitis fail conventional therapy and highlights treatment options useful in the palliative treatment of these patients.

Recent advancements in skull base surgery to remove or diminish the size of cranial base tumors allow more to be done than ever before to preserve life for patients who have tumors in anatomic locations once considered unreachable without causing massive functional impairment or death. Nonetheless, the resulting outcome has a direct and serious impact on the quality of life of the patient. In this article on palliation, the authors focus on the rehabilitative techniques used in patients who have undergone extensive cranial base resection. These techniques can also be used to improve the life of patients who have not undergone surgery but suffer from poor quality of life because of the natural growth of the tumor.

Recurrent respiratory papillomatosis (RRP) is a chronic, frequently debilitating, and potentially life-threatening disease. Therapy for RRP has evolved from simply inserting a tracheotomy to provide an airway and plucking out papillomata with cup forceps to provide some degree of voice to the present-day far more sophisticated approaches, along with preventative measures that may someday offer the potential dramatically to decrease disease prevalence. Family dynamics and support and intentional structuring of office protocols to accommodate the unique nature of RRP are as essential as any operative intervention for saving and prolonging life. This article reviews recent developments in the management of RRP and highlights palliative approaches to case management for those patients who are not easily cured with initial endoscopic interventions.

This article reviews the authors' work, which expands on previous studies to confirm that anxiety-related processes cause or maintain symptoms of dizziness. Discussed are interventions directed at patients' underlying psychologic disorders, including current methods of pharmacotherapy and psychotherapy. Patients with chronic complaints of nonspecific dizziness can present frustrating diagnostic and therapeutic challenges, but can be offered definitive and palliative care. The authors emphasize the importance of eliciting a precise description of the dizziness sensation from the patient as the critical factor in delineating the specific diagnosis and guiding treatment.

For physicians treating patients with sensorineural hearing loss, therapy is directed more toward helping the patient cope with the loss of hearing rather than offering various medical or surgical interventions. Accordingly, for the patient with sensorineural hearing loss, the care plan is usually more directed toward palliation than toward cure. This article views hearing loss not only as a physiologic deficit, but as the loss of an important aspect of overall communication skill that can have far reaching emotional and psychologic effects on the patient, the family, and those who surround patients in their daily lives. In this article the authors offer strategies for managing the patient who is losing or who has lost hearing.

This article defines palliative care for swallowing disorders as treatment for severe and chronic dysphagia or intractable aspiration when the recovery of normal swallowing is not anticipated and attempts to restore normal swallowing have been unsuccessful. Palliative treatment for dysphagia is not only for the dying patient because patients with difficulty swallowing can live for a long time. Palliative care for dysphagia is aimed at maximizing swallowing function, maintaining pulmonary health, and supporting healthy nutrition despite the impaired ability to swallow. When despite all attempts at intervention a patient becomes totally unable to swallow, the goal of therapy changes toward finding ways to provide adequate nutrition for the patient.

THE CLINICS ARE NOW AVAILABLE ONLINE!

Access your subscription at:
www.theclinics.com

Preface

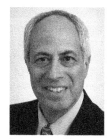 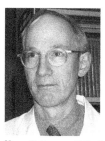

Kenneth M. Grundfast, MD, FACS   Geoffrey P. Dunn, MD, FACS
Guest Editors

AN OTOLARYNGOLOGIST WITH AN INTEREST IN PALLIATIVE CARE

Otolaryngologists do not ordinarily think of themselves as providers of palliative care. This may be more related to how we think about what we do rather than to the current existing and widely accepted concept of what actually constitutes palliative care. In this edition of the *Otolaryngology Clinics of North America*, the scope of palliative care is viewed as being far wider than simply care for the dying patient. In the last few decades, while the scope of otolaryngology–head and neck surgery has been widening significantly, the scope of palliative care has become continually more expansive, and *palliative medicine* has become now a distinct medical specialty officially recognized by the American Board of Medical Specialties.

For sure, a delightful aspect of practicing otolaryngology–head and neck surgery flows from the sense that so many patients seeking otolaryngic care can benefit greatly from the array of medical and surgical interventions that we have to offer. The applications of laser technology, the advent of cochlear implants, the ability to do sinus surgery using endoscopes, and new minimally invasive approaches to neck surgery, including thyroidectomy, along with the concomitant continual introduction of newer and more effective medications, has enabled the otolaryngologist of today to do more than ever before to help patients with otolaryngic disorders, including those with cancer of the head and neck. Certainly, restoring normal hearing with a stapedectomy must be one of the most rewarding experiences any surgeon can have. Similarly, inserting a cochlear implant and watching a deaf patient hear again or watching a congenitally deaf child hear for the first time can be an exhilarating experience for both the patient and his or her physician. Excising a cancerous oral cavity lesion and artfully reconstructing the surgical defect is both challenging and deeply satisfying especially when the outcome for the patient appears to be good. Even simply removing nasal polyps, inserting tubes in a child's ears, and removing tonsils and adenoids can make the kinds of differences in the lives of patients that give the surgeon a great sense of accomplishment. Thus, in general, otolaryngologists become accustomed to helping patients, often quickly seeing the tangible benefits of their work perhaps in an

Otolaryngol Clin N Am 42 (2009) xiii–xvi
doi:10.1016/j.otc.2008.09.014
0030-6665/08/$ – see front matter © 2009 Elsevier Inc. All rights reserved.

improved audiogram, an improved postoperative sinus computed tomography scan, or in declaring a patient cured of cancer many years after an extirpative surgery. Nonetheless, every otolaryngologist knows that not all patients improve after a specific medical therapy has been tried or surgery has been done. We have successes, and we also encounter frustrations when patients continue to have troublesome symptoms despite having received treatment. Although we have become accustomed to seeing the successful outcome of the treatments we routinely provide, every experienced otolaryngologist knows that our scope of practice includes the management of disorders for which there really is no universally effective treatment, and some of our patients with cancer will not survive despite our valiant efforts.

This edition of the *Otolaryngology Clinics of North America* has been prepared to provide information on how to manage those patients who have otolaryngic disorders that cannot be completely fixed, eradicated, or cured. The purpose of providing the information in this edition is to enlighten the otolaryngologist about how to care for patients for whom medical or surgical management cannot totally alleviate symptoms or achieve a cure. After all, we have to admit to ourselves and to our patients that we do not have a cure for tinnitus nor can we stop the progressive hearing loss that we define as presbycusis. Even though we do endoscopic sinus surgery, many patients with chronic sinus disease continue to have nasal obstruction and rhinorrhea after surgery, and some patients who have had excision of cancer of the head and neck have persistent or recurrent disease. In this volume, the reader will learn how those who have experience with various aspects of otolaryngology deal with the patients who need medical management directed at minimizing symptoms, coping with chronic conditions, and alleviating pain and suffering rather than aiming for complete cure. Palliative care has become a distinct medical subspecialty, and the time has come for otolaryngologists to know about the aspects of palliative care that are pertinent to the practice of otolaryngology–head and neck surgery.

Kenneth M. Grundfast, MD, FACS
Department of Otolaryngology–Head and Neck Surgery
Boston University School of Medicine
Boston Medical Center
Office of Student Affairs
Boston University School of Medicine
830 Harrison Avenue
Boston, MA 02118, USA

A SURGEON NOW BOARD CERTIFIED IN PALLIATIVE CARE

I am often asked, "How did you, a surgeon, become interested in palliative care?" There were many beginnings to my work in hospice and palliative care that occurred during my training and earlier surgical practice that I never appreciated until recently. Time has allowed me to see increasingly more the fundamental similarities of surgical and palliative care instead of the distracting and more superficial differences. Years before I had heard of palliative care or had any direct contact with hospice patients, I was involved in the care of patients with progressive, incurable, and life-limiting illness. In many of these cases, such as in trauma and critical care, the circumstances were acute and required immediate and decisive intervention. Like most surgeons and surgeons-in-training, I was proud of the expediency and effectiveness with which I could intervene on a patient's behalf in life-threatening situations; however, I felt equally fulfilled on occasions when comforting a distressed patient, whether reassuring a young woman with a fibroadenoma of the breast or counseling a cancer patient facing approaching and unavoidable demise. I learned from fatally burned patients, geriatric patients with overwhelming abdominal sepsis, and infants with catastrophic congenital anomalies and neonatal conditions that hoping for a good prognosis or intervening to improve it was too-limiting a perspective for much of the spectrum of surgical care. Saving life and saving hope are no longer synonymous in a time when the definition of life, itself, has become so biologically, socially, and spiritually complex. Saving life is not necessary for the salvation of hope as long as hope, itself, can be redefined. Closely related to the preservation of hope is the cardinal principal of nonabandonment. Surgeons have always enjoyed the moral pride that comes by standing in the patient's corner when all seemed lost to the patient, his family, and even our colleagues. I believe it is the premier value we as surgeons place upon the virtue of nonabandonment that makes palliative care so relevant to us and makes it so fitting that we become more active in its development as a medical field.

I believe that a fundamental shift in our orientation to the focus of care will be necessary to extend the reach of surgical care to the complete spectrum of illness. In fact, the treatment of illness rather than disease is the point of departure from the traditional biophysical model of orientation of care to organ systems. Disease occurs in organs; illness, which is the individual's experience of disease, occurs in people. Should the shift in orientation from disease to illness occur, head and neck surgeons of the future may join the fortunate ones of the past and present to see themselves more broadly as specialists in the care of persons afflicted with diseases of the head and neck, instead of mere specialists in the surgical treatment of diseases of the head and neck.

Ten years ago, when sharing my accumulating experience in hospice and palliative care with fellow surgeons and surgical residents, I recognized that transforming surgery from treatment of disease to the treatment of illness would be as daunting a task as surgeons overcoming avoidance or outright denial of death in their practices.

It seemed ironic to me when a surgeon who encountered death in patients from trauma on at least a weekly basis told me once "I can't imagine how you can deal with death and dying." The uneasiness of surgeons' acceptance of the patient-centered (illness, not disease, orientation) approach to care and the acceptance of death as a natural sequel and precursor to life are the two main psychological barriers to their unconditional acceptance of palliative care as an essential component of surgical care.

The American Board of Surgery was one of the sponsoring boards of the American Board of Medical Specialties' (ABMS) newly formed Board of Hospice and Palliative Medicine. The first certifying examination of the new board will be given in October 2008. Through the American Board of Surgery, otolaryngologists can seek ABMS certification in hospice and palliative medicine. Even if the number of potentially interested otolaryngologists is quite small, the potential impact of this group could be considerable given the early stage of evolution the field and the growing general interest in quality-of-life outcomes in surgical practice. I was certified by the previous American Board of Hospice and Palliative Medicine during its first year of certifying exams in 1997 with another surgeon, Robert Milch, who pioneered hospice care in Buffalo as early as the late 1970s. Other surgeons have since been certified, and awareness and interest in palliative care by surgeons has been documented in several studies.

Expanding our horizon for care will require new self-awareness, new language, and new skills, starting with the ability to communicate with patients in situations in which we had previously dreaded having to say anything. I have always believed that what we now describe as palliative care is not an exotic new idea, but it is an approach that has always been consistent with good surgical care. Recent attention to the compelling needs of the most desperately and terminally ill has only highlighted the many unanswered needs of all patients. In time, the current period of growth in the field of palliative care may be looked back upon as the beginning (or return ?) of a more humane vision of *all* patient care. How ironic that the care of the hopeless and the previously abandoned could become the moral and scientific basis for the salvation of the soul and future of all surgery itself!

Geoffrey P. Dunn, MD, FACS
Department of Surgery
Palliative Care Consultation Service
Hamot Medical Center
201 State Street
Erie, PA 16550, USA

Dedication

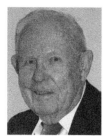

Dr. Pratt

This volume is dedicated to the venerable and distinguished Dr. Loring Pratt of Waterville, Maine who has had an illustrious career as an otolaryngologist. Dr. Pratt has served as Regent of the American College of Surgeons, First President of the American Academy of Otolaryngology–Head and Neck Surgery (AAO-HNS), Chair of the AAO-HNS Ethics Committee, and Chair of the AAO-HNS History and Archives Committee.

Dr. Pratt accomplished all of this while also being father to nine children, grandfather to 26 children, devoted husband, avid amateur photographer and botanist, and student of medical history. He has been a mentor to many and a loyal friend—in many ways he is what all physicians strive to be. In a sense, Dr. Pratt was providing compassionate care and palliative care to patients throughout Maine before the world of medicine knew much about what we now view as the distinct specialty of palliative medicine. We are indebted to Dr. Pratt and therefore dedicate this volume to him in recognition of his years of leadership and his endless willingness to help others.

Ken Grundfast

Geoff Dunn

Otolaryngol Clin N Am 42 (2009) xvii
doi:10.1016/j.otc.2008.09.015
0030-6665/08/$ – see front matter © 2009 Elsevier Inc. All rights reserved.

oto.theclinics.com

Principles and Core Competencies of Surgical Palliative Care: an Overview

Geoffrey P. Dunn, MD, FACS

KEYWORDS

• Surgical palliative care • Palliative care • Palliative surgery

The experience and success of the hospice movement in the United States and abroad was followed by the extension of its basic concepts to the much larger population of patients with advanced, but not necessarily terminal, illness. This collective experience has provided the necessary background and stimulus for developing a specific set of principles and competencies applicable to surgical palliative care that includes surgery of the head and neck.

The National Consensus Project for Quality Palliative Care, representing a coalition of the American Academy of Hospice and Palliative Care, the Hospice and Palliative Nurses Association, and the National Hospice and Palliative Care Organization, outlined the domains and structures of high quality palliative care.[1] By these guidelines, the competent medical practitioner in conjunction with a palliative care team ensures the following: expert pain and nonpain symptom control is addressed with patients and families throughout the course of illness in a coordinated manner across settings; information and news are communicated in a timely, sensitive, comprehensible manner respecting treatment goals; care is reassessed and coordinated across settings in the context of a trusting patient-practitioner relationship; and opportunity is given for preparation for the dying process and death as well as support for growth and bereavement.

The American College of Surgeons has, over the course of 10 years, developed its own principles of palliative care, commencing with the article "Principles Guiding Care at End of Life"[2] as the national debate about physician-assisted suicide had reached fever pitch. Subsequently, its current "Statement of Principles of Palliative Care"[3] (**Box 1**) was endorsed when it was recognized that palliative care is equally appropriate to patients earlier in the course of illness, including those receiving life-prolonging treatments.

Palliative Care, Hamot Medical Center, 201 State Street, Erie, PA 16550, USA
E-mail address: gpdunn1@earthlink.net

Otolaryngol Clin N Am 42 (2009) 1–13
doi:10.1016/j.otc.2008.09.003
0030-6665/08/$ – see front matter © 2009 Elsevier Inc. All rights reserved.

Box 1
American College of Surgeons statement of principles of palliative care

- Respect the dignity and autonomy of patients, patients' surrogates, and caregivers.
- Honor the right of the competent patient or surrogate to choose among treatments, including those that may or may not prolong life.
- Communicate effectively and empathically with patients, their families, and caregivers.
- Identify the primary goals of care from the patient's perspective and address how the surgeon's care can achieve the patient's objectives.
- Strive to alleviate pain and other burdensome physical and nonphysical symptoms.
- Recognize, assess, discuss, and offer access to services for psychologic, social, and spiritual issues.
- Provide access to therapeutic support, encompassing the spectrum from life-prolonging treatments through hospice care, when they can realistically be expected to improve the quality of life as perceived by the patient.
- Recognize the physician's responsibility to discourage treatments that are unlikely to achieve the patient's goals and encourage patients and families to consider hospice care when the prognosis for survival is likely to be less than a half-year.
- Arrange for continuity of care by the patient's primary or specialist physician, alleviating the sense of abandonment patients may feel when "curative" therapies are no longer useful.
- Maintain a collegial and supportive attitude toward others entrusted with care of the patient.

From Task Force on Surgical Palliative care; Committee on Ethics. Statement of principles of palliative care. Bull Am Coll Surg 2005;90(8):34–5; with permission.

The practice of surgical palliative care is, at the least, a fundamental component of good surgical clinical care and, at most, the foundation of all surgical care. The relief of suffering and the maintenance of quality of life are outcomes surgeons should strive for in all patients, not just those clearly at the end of their lives. To achieve this, the minimum expected of all surgeons regardless of their specialty are competence in providing palliation concurrently with curative treatment, the ability to gently transition from one of these approaches to the other, and the provision of procedural skills for which the surgeon is qualified to palliate as well as to cure. Achieving these outcomes presumes, as unfunded mandates frequently do, considerable flexibility on the part of the surgeon who has typically not had the benefit of formal training in communication of bad news, effective pain and nonpain symptom management,[4] or the support of a culture that consistently prioritizes survival and cure over the relief of patient suffering or emphasizes achievement of physician-defined goals.

The Accreditation Council on Graduate Medical Education (ACGME) has identified six core competencies expected of a qualified surgeon:

1. patient care
2. medical knowledge
3. practice-based learning and improvement
4. interpersonal and communication skills
5. professionalism and
6. systems-based practice

The core competencies are now the required framework for curricula of all ACGME-accredited surgical residencies. The Surgical Palliative Care Task Force of the

American College of Surgeons has identified specific competencies for palliative care using the ACGME core competency model (**Box 2**).[5]

PATIENT CARE: A CORE COMPETENCY FOR SURGICAL PALLIATIVE CARE

The salient issues and practices for surgical palliative care are addressed herein using the heading of "Patient care" from the outline of core competencies identified by the Surgical Palliative Care Task Force of the American College of Surgeons.

"Possess the capacity to guide the transition from curative and palliative goals of treatment to palliative goals alone based on patient information and preferences, scientific and outcomes evidence, and sound clinical judgment."

The barriers to transition from curative to palliative goals are similar to the barriers already identified in achieving effective pain control. They consist of the practitioner's cognitive gaps and attitudes, socioeconomic realities, and cultural differences. These barriers are not all imposed by the practitioner or the medical care system. A noncompliant patient reporting poor pain relief despite having a valid and appropriate unfilled prescription in hand or a family's insistence on pursuing unrealistic treatments point to other barriers that should be considered as some of the etiologies for unrelieved pain. Overcoming these barriers requires the practitioner to genuinely believe that the relief of suffering is a concurrent, not a subservient, goal to the preservation or prolongation of life.

Palliation is, fundamentally, a moral calling. If the willingness to alleviate suffering is present, success can follow because the necessary evidence base for many effective interventions is present and growing. The skills required to relieve suffering, such as pain management and the empathic response, can be learned. Sound clinical judgment in palliative care is no different than in other venues. It assumes the capacity to never make some types of mistakes and to make the remainder infrequently.

"Perform an assessment and gather essential clinical information about symptoms, pain, and suffering."

Patient assessment for palliative care or "seeing the big picture" addresses four dimensions of the patient's experience: physical, emotional (psychologic), social (economic), and spiritual (existential). The American Medical Association sponsored Education of Physicians on End-of-Life Care (EPEC) curriculum designates nine domains of interest (**Box 3**) when performing an assessment, although all of these domains are not always addressed or appropriate to address. Palliative care assessment is not only an intervention that helps establish trust but also provides the opportunity for triage. Unrelieved somatic pain rating 8 out of 10 in intensity needs to be addressed before addressing spiritual needs even if these are ultimately more important to the patient. Over the course of a series of conversations, all of the relevant domains can be assessed in a relaxed fashion by the surgeon or other members of the interdisciplinary team. Palliative care assessment forms[6] and scoring systems are available, although development of a palliative care assessment specific for the field of otolaryngology remains an opportunity. Validated tools specific for the assessment of pain[7] and nonpain symptoms (dyspnea,[8] depression[9]), which are part of the overall palliative care assessment, are available.

"Perform palliative procedures competently and with sound judgment to meet patient goals of care at the end of life."

Box 2
Core competencies for surgical palliative care

Patient care

- Possess the capacity to guide the transition from curative and palliative goals of treatment to palliative goals alone based on patient information and preferences, scientific and outcomes evidence, and sound clinical judgment.

- Perform an assessment and gather essential clinical information about symptoms, pain, and suffering.

- Perform palliative procedures competently and with sound judgment to meet patient goals of care at the end of life.

- Provide management of pain and other symptoms to alleviate suffering.

- Communicate effectively and compassionately bad news and poor prognoses.

- Conduct a patient and family meeting regarding advance directives and end-of-life decisions.

- Exercise sound clinical judgment and skill in the withdrawal and withholding of life support.

Medical knowledge

Surgeons should acquire knowledge in the fundamentals of palliative care applicable to the breadth of their surgical patients. These fundamentals include the following:

- Acute and chronic pain management

- Nonpain symptom management

- Ethical and legal basis for advance directives, informed consent, withdrawal and withholding of life support, and futility

- Grief and bereavement in surgical illness

- Quality of life outcomes and prognostication

- Role of spirituality at the end of life

Practice-based learning and improvement

- Recognize quality of life and quality of death and dying outcomes as important components of the morbidity and mortality review process.

- Understand their measurement and integration into peer review process and quality improvement of practice.

- Be skilled in the use of introspection and self-monitoring for practice improvement.

Interpersonal and communication skills

Surgeons must be competent and compassionate communicators with patients, families, and other health care providers. They should be effective in communicating bad news and prognosis and in redefining hope in the context of cultural diversity. The interdisciplinary nature of palliative care requires that the surgeon is skilled as a leader and a member of an interdisciplinary team and maintains collegial relationships with other health care providers.

Professionalism

Surgeons must maintain a professional commitment to ethical and empathic care that is patient focused, with equal attention to relief of suffering along with curative therapy. Respect and compassion for cultural diversity, gender, and disability is particularly important around rituals and bereavement at the end of life. Maintenance of ethical standards in the withholding and withdrawal of life support is essential.

Systems-based practice

Surgeons must be aware and informed of the multiple components of the health care system that provide palliative and end-of-life care. Surgeons should be knowledgeable and willing to refer patients to resources such as hospice, palliative care consultation, pain management, pastoral care, and social services and should understand the resource use and reimbursement issues involved.

Adapted from Office of Promoting Excellence in End-of-Life Care: Surgeons' Palliative Care Workgroup Report from the Field. J Am Coll Surg 2003;197(4):661–85; with permission.

Box 3
EPEC's nine dimensions of whole patient assessment for palliative care

1. Illness/treatment summary

2. Physical

3. Psychologic

4. Decision making

5. Communication

6. Social

7. Spiritual

8. Practical

9. Anticipatory planning for death

From Whole patient assessment. In: EPEC Project, American Medical Association. Trainers's guide. Chicago: American Medical Association; 1999; with permission.

"Provide management of pain and other symptoms to alleviate suffering."
"Communicate bad news and poor prognoses effectively and compassionately."

A narrative abstracted from my practice experience demonstrates these patient care competencies. A 54-year-old unemployed divorced man with a 60-pack per year smoking history presented to the emergency room with a several month history of left-sided neck pain, dysphagia, and a 40-pound weight loss. His pain was self-described as constant, aching, and burning. He reported minimal relief with acetaminophen and hydrocodone that had been previously prescribed for dental problems. On physical examination, he appeared to be an older middle-aged man with pallor and temporal wasting. His affect was flat, although he appeared apprehensive with minimal physical exertion. Respirations were 40 per minute, shallow, and stridorous. Bulky, hard, confluent adenopathy of the left side of the neck was present. Oral examination was limited due to marked trismus. The hematocrit was 32, serum albumin 2.5, and total protein 5.4 g/L. In the emergency room, he uttered, "I can't breathe... pain...getting worse. Please...do what you need to do...." Following informed consent, he was promptly taken to the operating room where urgent tracheostomy was performed. Further evaluation of the oral cavity under general anesthesia revealed poor dentition and a large fungating mass extending from the nasopharynx down to the vallecula. A biopsy of the mass and a feeding gastrostomy were performed. Biopsy demonstrated poorly differentiated, keratinizing, squamous cell carcinoma. Chest CT showed multiple nodules consistent with metastases.

On the first postoperative day he was clinically stable and had tube feedings initiated. Consultation was sought from medical and radiation oncologists, although the patient adamantly declined these interventions, saying he "just wanted to go home." The attending surgeon, exasperated with the patient's therapeutic nihilism, consulted the palliative care service to "get a DNR order and get hospice involved."

During the initial interview, the patient was alert and oriented. He complained (when asked) of pain in the left side of the neck and upper abdomen with an intensity of 8 on a scale of 10. He had been declining his prescribed analgesic of oxycodone, 10 mg per percutaneous endoscopic gastrostomy tube every 4 hours. On examination, his brow was furrowed, respirations were 28 per minute and shallow, and his abdomen was flat and tense with occasional bowel sounds. The tracheostomy and gastrostomy were functioning. Accompanying him was his live-in companion of several years. The patient gave his preference and permission to discuss his care with her separately. Before this interview, he was persuaded to take his analgesic to "lessen his shortness of breath and overall discomfort" and was told we would return soon to review our discussion if he wished.

During the interview with the patient's companion, she commenced speaking with a burst of tears and then gave a narrative of the past several months during which time the patient had become increasingly symptomatic but refused seeking medical care because of a lack of insurance and, she suspected, the fear of confirming the presence of cancer. He attributed his symptoms to ongoing dental problems. He had tried a succession of "alternative" remedies for his swelling in addition to gargling with mouthwash. His pain had led him to try ice packs, heat, and old pain prescriptions. After he had lost considerable weight, he became more depressed and had talked about "wanting to end it all." Witnessing this, she said she felt helpless, exhausted, and "at wit's end." She acknowledged feeling calmer now that he was under medical care, although she described herself as "still in a state of shock." When asked what she knew of his condition, she responded, "I know he has cancer of the neck, but not much more than that." When asked if she wanted to know more details about its stage and prognosis, she said she was unsure. After telling her that that information would be available when she wished to have it, the discussion was then directed to assessing the patient's family support, spiritual history, economic situation, and the immediate strategy to improve his physical and mental comfort.

Upon seeing her companion more relaxed after this discussion, she, now more composed and hopeful, asked for information about his disease and its prognosis. In the presence of his nurse and with a box of tissue paper nearby, she confirmed she preferred direct nonmedical terminology. She was given information building on the fact that she already was aware he had cancer, "You mentioned your partner has cancer of the neck. That much we know is true, as confirmed by the biopsy that was just done. When we want to determine the extent of cancer, we stage it. The stage of the cancer is a guide for its prognosis and treatment. Unfortunately, your partner's cancer is in its most advanced stage and is not curable at this point." The patient's partner, tearful and looking down, shook her head in acknowledgment. After a silent pause, the surgeon stated as he offered her a tissue, "I can see how distressing this news is for you, even though you may have suspected this." She nodded affirmatively again and then looking directly at the surgeon asked, "How much time does he have?" The surgeon responded, "That depends on several things—some under our control, others not. His decisions about the type of treatment could impact survival, though unforeseen events such as infection could lessen his time of survival, even if treated. Untreated for cancer he is unlikely to survive beyond several months, especially if he declines tube feeding or forced hydration in the near future. Exceptions to the usual course of untreated disease of this extent are exceptional. We can't be sure exactly how his course will run, but I can be sure we will be there to help you, regardless of the type of treatment he selects." Imploringly she asked, "What do we do now?" The surgeon responded, "Let's see if he is comfortable, first. He may want to rest right now, but I will ask him if he would like to know what we discussed. If he wants to know, I will ask him what I asked you: When would he like to talk about it and in how much detail? If he just wants to rest after the ordeal of the past day (and weeks), we will arrange a time at his convenience and, in the meantime, you can reach me with questions at this number [card given]."

"Conduct a patient and family meeting regarding advance directives and end-of-life decisions."

The family meeting is a critical tool for effective palliative care, whether conveying adverse news, resolving conflict, or determining goals of care. Scheduled family meetings for determination of care goals have been shown to result in several favorable outcomes, among them reduced length of ICU admissions[10,11] and increased rates of organ donation.[12] General guidelines for a family meeting recommend a previously agreed upon agenda, punctuality, privacy, adequate seating, nonintrusion by pagers, a facilitator for discussion, and a professional medical translator when needed. The subject of advance directives or a "living will" and "do not resuscitate" (DNR) order may be broached but should only be done so after gentle probing for the degree of insight of the patient and family and establishing a relaxed context for asking about specific medical preferences. This discussion may proceed by asking, "Have you ever had a chance to discuss (eg, with your wife or a family member) what your preferences for medical treatment are in the event of a serious or life-limiting illness? Many people have not discussed these matters because this sounds frightening, but not as frightening as leaving these decisions to chance. If you couldn't tell us yourself for some reason, whom would you designate to speak on your behalf? Some people have answers to these questions in what is referred to as a 'living will' or 'advance directives.' Do you have one?"

A well-conducted family meeting or patient interview during which unwelcome news is disclosed can be as rewarding an experience to the surgeon as any well-done invasive procedure. Clinical communication is an invasive procedure. Badly conveyed information can have a lasting impact on families, even manifesting itself later as posttraumatic stress disorder in some instances.[13] The operation is a reassuring metaphor for surgeons who may be uneasy when giving bad news, because communication, like surgery, can be learned with good mentoring.

"Exercise sound clinical judgment and skill in the withdrawal and withholding of life support."

The process of withdrawal or withholding of life support requires a knowledge base and group of skills consisting of prognostication, familiarity with the moral, ethical, and legal basis for withholding or withdrawing medical treatment, communication of anticipated physiologic changes and their implications for palliative interventions, and the ability to intervene promptly and effectively.

When life-prolonging or invasive treatments become doubtful means of achieving a patient's goals of care, the option of withdrawal or withholding them should be discussed.

Although head and neck surgeons may only rarely be directly involved in this type of discussion, they may serve as consultants to patients in the critical care setting in which this type of decision making is a daily occurrence. For surgeons managing patients with head and neck tumors, an empathic discussion about the normal trajectory of disease untreated or unresponsive to treatment and knowledge of what can be done to mitigate suffering in all its forms as a consequence of this are more reliable ways to preserve a patient's hope than nondisclosure or detached referral. The support of the consulting surgeon can be invaluable in validating complicated medical decisions, especially those that direct life support to be withheld or withdrawn. Familiarity with the current consensus of medical ethicists and landmark US judicial opinions[14–18] of the past 3 decades are helpful in discussing the difference between "killing" or "playing God" and allowing natural death. Occasionally, it is helpful to remind surrogates that, from legal and ethical perspectives, the decision to withdraw a treatment is the same as never having started it.

Ventilator support is the most obvious example of the group of treatments collectively known as life support. When tracheostomy for ongoing ventilator support is being considered instead of discontinuation of ventilator support, the surgeon should be aware of the approach and technique of ventilator withdrawal to provide a more complete context for the informed consent process and to better support individuals who make the weighty decision to decline further life support measures.

The decision to withdraw ventilator support can be extremely difficult for surrogates even when the patient may have designated this wish in an advance directive and the surrogate completely agrees. This difficulty is usually due to the following:

1. doubt about the given prognosis for recovery
2. fear that withdrawal will lead to physical suffering and
3. fear that making this decision is tantamount to killing the patient. No one is better positioned to authoritatively dispel these doubts and fears than the concerned physician, even if additional reassurance is needed from a professional with sophisticated knowledge of the relevant law and ethics or an individual entrusted with the spiritual care for the individual.

Prognostication, once the most valued skill of medical practitioners, is making a comeback in its clinical importance because of improvements in disease staging, experience with functional assessment scales such as the Karnofsky Performance Scale, and the recognition that accurate prognostication enhances patient autonomy. The rewards of accurate prognostication and the penalty paid for not prognosticating are the main reasons for the reestablishment of its importance in patient goal-oriented care. The functional status of the patient is the single most reliable predictor of prognosis.[19] The Palliative Performance Scale (PPS)[20] is a validated, observer-rated scale that correlates ambulation, activity level, extent of clinical disease, self-care, intake by mouth, and level of consciousness with the Karnofsky scale, which allows correlation of these domains with actual and median survival. The PPS has been validated for cancer patients admitted for inpatient hospice or palliative care. A PPS score of 50% correlates with a patient who mainly sits or lies, requires considerable assistance, and has normal to reduced intake. Confusion not related to a specific central nervous system lesion but stemming from general debility may be evident. At a 50% score, extensive disease is present, and the estimated life expectancy is in the range of 2 to 4 weeks.[21,22]

Explanation of the physiologic basis for the predictable efficacy of medications used to prevent dyspnea, anxiety, and excessive secretions is one of the most effective means of allaying the fear that the patient will suffer following extubation. It is important to explain that the purpose of medications used in this situation is to relieve symptoms and not hasten demise. It is also important to explain to the family that death does not necessarily immediately follow extubation of patients who are able to breathe independently. This discussion should be documented.

Death can promptly follow cessation of ventilator support because of cardiopulmonary arrest due to hypoxia or hypercarbia from respiratory failure, although the medications given before extubation may appear to be the direct (and intentional) cause of death. Paralytic agents have no place in the process of ventilator support withdrawal because their use would hasten death without any favorable impact on the symptoms associated with withdrawal of ventilator support. The principle of double effect is the ethical framework within which the potential undesired effects of medication (including the hastening of death) are acceptable if the intention of their use is the relief of suffering,[23] although it has been shown that sedative dose increases in the last week and hours of life are not associated with shortened survival when compared with withholding such sedation. The use of deliberate sedation for the relief of intractable symptoms does not shorten survival when these patients are compared with those who do not receive such sedation during the last days of life in hospice care.[24,25]

Two general approaches to ventilator withdrawal are used—immediate extubation and terminal weaning.

Two approaches to ventilator withdrawal are used when ventilator support remains necessary for survival but is no longer desired as a treatment: 1) Immediate extubation; 2) Terminal weaning.

Immediate Extubation

For immediate extubation (usually the preferred approach), the endotracheal tube is removed after appropriate endotracheal suction and pre-medication with opioids (2-10 mg morphine intravenously and anxioloytics midazolam 1 to 2 mg IV or lorazepam 1-2 mg IV).[26] If more copious secretions are anticipated, anti-secretory medication (glycopyrrolate) is administered. Occasionally stridor occurs following extubation. This should be treated promptly with inhaled racemic epinephrine and intravenous dexamethasone. Patients with considerable volume overload are more likely to have noisy breathing from copious secretions after extubation and family should be counseled that noisy breathing due to upper airway secretions is not "drowning." I have found that families are less apprehensive about extubation under these circumstances when they are told that this is the procedure that is followed when removing the tube after a general anesthetic. A physician experienced in ventilator withdrawal should be present during and in the immediate aftermath of extubation, not only because complications (eg, refractory agitation, stridor) can develop quickly and need to be treated quickly, but also because of the added reassurance this brings to understandably anxious family members.

Terminal Weaning

Occasionally, terminal weaning is the preferred method of ventilator withdrawal, such as in apneic patients, patients with threatened airway obstruction, or those with copious secretions. Using this approach, the ventilator settings are tapered down over an hour or longer, leaving the endotracheal tube in. The ventilator, when weaned down, can be disconnected and removed from the room leaving the endotracheal tube in with a T-piece.

Extubation Follow-Through

Family should be given the chance to prepare themselves prior to ventilator withdrawal and they should be given the option to be present during and after extubation. These preparations may involve the presence of the family's chaplain, the arrival of others who would want to be present, and arrangements for rituals and music. A gesture as simple as asking a family member if their dying loved one would like to have a keepsake from home, such as a quilt, creates a context for this experience that goes far beyond simply meeting medical needs. The room should be cleared of medical impedimenta and other devices (nasogastric tubes, sequential leg compression devices) not relevant to patient comfort. Monitors should be silenced and removed when possible to prevent unnecessary distraction or family misinterpretation of the various tracings. Venous access should be maintained along with ready-to-administer additional sedative and opioid.

Following extubation, additional medication should be titrated to the patient's symptoms. Privacy for the family should be balanced with frequent reassessment of the patient's condition and symptom control. Opioids and sedatives should be available on a sub-hourly PRN basis in addition to any basal hourly infusions of these that may be running. Should the patient survive, he or she should remain in the unit for at least several hours to assure durable and predictable control of symptoms before transferring to a general floor. In instances of prolonged survival, discussion with family should broach possible discharge to a nursing facility or home with hospice follow-up.

The physician should be mindful that the process of ventilator withdrawal not only has an emotional impact on family, but also nurses, respiratory therapists, and others working closely with the patient. Acknowledging this impact either in the course of informal follow-up contact or more formal meetings may be helpful in identifying or mitigating "burnout" while offering the physician a reality check by colleagues about the status of his own psyche. Despite the sadness of the undertaking, when compassionately and competently done, the appropriate withdrawal of ventilator support is deeply appreciated by family members, making it among the most rewarding of clinical duties.

For situations in which there are actual or perceived ethical dilemmas about the choice or discontinuation of therapy at end of life, referral to a palliative care team is a more expedient and helpful source of guidance than an ethics committee referral, because a properly trained palliative care team should not only be well versed in the ethical issues related to withholding or withdrawal of care, but also have the expertise to communicate effectively with patients and families in addition to managing distressing symptoms. In hospitals that have both palliative care consultation services and an ethics committee, the ethics committee's deliberations on cases related to end-of-life care should be reserved for reviewing treatment protocols, arbitration in instances of intractable conflict between patient/family and health care providers not resolved by the palliative care team, and review of ethical concerns involving the palliative care team, itself.

OTHER TOOLS FOR SURGICAL PALLIATIVE CARE
Palliative Surgery

Palliative surgery is one of the principle tools of surgical palliative care. It has been defined as "any invasive procedure in which the main intention is to mitigate physical symptoms in patients with non-curable disease without causing premature death."[27] Earlier definitions have been problematic when applied to the current concept of palliative care because they were based upon their impact (or lack of it) upon *disease*, rather than symptoms, such as when used to describe procedures resulting in tumor-positive tissue margins or recurrence. Hofmann et al. point out that the difficulty of defining palliative surgery lies in epistemological and ethical considerations. Under no other circumstances is informed consent more critical because of the physical and psychologic vulnerability of this patient population. Future research will require much more attention to quality of life outcomes measures in addition to the traditional measures of mortality and morbidity. The Division of Surgery under the chairmanship of Lawrence D. Wagman has successfully and prolifically pioneered the concept of palliative surgery as an interdisciplinary process consistent with evidence-based palliative care as it is evolving in this country.[28] No other group has done more to highlight the differences between a non-curative operation and a palliative one, a difference that has yet to be more clearly determined by all surgeons of all subspecialties.

Systems-Based Practice

A surgeon can greatly extend his impact in providing and improving palliative care by willingness to refer to widely available resources. Barriers to good palliative care frequently stem from the surgeon's unwillingness to acknowledge the advanced stage of the patient's illness. Fear of "taking away hope" is a frequent reason why limited prognosis and the implicitly appropriate management are not initiated sooner by the surgeon. Not infrequently, colleagues tell me that a patient or family is "not ready" for palliative care or hospice. Almost invariably, this is more a reflection of the surgeon's uneasiness with the evolving clinical situation and what it implies for medical guidance (which he may not be able to confidently provide) than a reflection of the family's wishes. Part of the palliative care team's training is how to approach the patient who is not ready. Good communication and symptom control are never too soon and it is exceedingly rare for a family to regret having palliative care expertise at their disposal as long as it is not naively presented to them as less care or a "hands off" approach. With respect to physicians' role in palliative care for patients, Lee Iaccoca's memorable advice applies: "Lead, follow, or get out of the way!"

The current array of palliative care resources for in- and outpatients includes hospice, palliative care teams, pain management consultation services, pastoral care services, ethics committees and social services. All of these services can be bundled in a palliative care or hospice team, while in many hospitals these needs are delegated separately. No diagnosis is excluded for referral to palliative care services as long as the illness is serious and life-limiting or potentially life-limiting. The criteria for Medicare Hospice Benefit (MHB) referral include: (1) eligibility for Part A of Medicare and (2) terminally ill with a life expectancy of 6 months or less if the disease runs its usual course. Certification by two physicians is required initially, then only one physician is required to certify for subsequent benefit periods. Most private insurers offer a hospice benefit with admission criteria similar to the MHB. An increasing number of hospice and home nursing programs are offering palliative care services for patients with a more lengthy prognosis or for patients not ready to commit to acceptance of the disease process without attempts to reverse or delay it.

CONCLUSION

By virtue of the many serious and life-limiting illnesses encountered by head and neck surgeons, opportunities are legion for the application of palliative care principles and competencies to clinical practice. Burdensome symptoms, patient communication difficulties, and ethical dilemmas unique to otolaryngology that would be best researched by head and neck surgeons now have a conceptual model of care that can build upon an interdisciplinary experience and evidence base that has been accumulating outside of the field of otolaryngology for several decades. For those inclined to pursue palliative care in more depth, hundreds of hospital and out-patient palliative care programs now exist which would welcome and cultivate the interest of a head and neck surgeon. For the rare few who are even more interested, the options of hospice and palliative medicine fellowship training and certification are available.

For the vast majority, however, the arrival of a systematic approach to the care of our most grievously afflicted patients will bring reassurance that our most basic impulse to relieve suffering will not find us wanting in responding in a way that is humane and helpful.

REFERENCES

1. National Consensus Project for Quality Palliative Care (2004). Clinical practice guidelines for quality palliative care. Available at: http://www.nationalconsensusproject. org. Accessed July 1, 2008.
2. Committee on Ethics, American College of Surgeons. Principles guiding care at end of life. Bull Am Coll Surg 1998;83:46.
3. Surgical Palliative Care Task Force, Committee of Ethics, American College of Surgeons. ACS statement of principles of palliative care. Bull Am Coll Surg 2005;90(8):34–5.
4. Galante JM, Bowles TL, Khatri VP, et al. Experience and attitudes of surgeons toward palliation in cancer. Arch Surg 2005;140(9):873–80.
5. Surgeons' Palliative Care Workgroup. Office of Promoting Excellence in End-of-Life Care: report from the field. J Am Coll Surg 2003;197(4):661–85.
6. Mularski RA, Osborne ML. Palliative care and intensive care unit care: preadmission assessment no. 122. J Palliat Med 2006;9(5):1204–5.
7. Jacox A, Carr DB, Payne R. Management of cancer pain: clinical practice guideline no. 9. AHCPR Publication no. 94-0592. Rockville (MD): Agency for Health Care Policy and Research, US Department of Health and Human Services, Public Health Service; 1994.
8. Bausewein C, Farquhar M, Booth S, et al. Measurement of breathlessness in advanced disease: a systematic review. Respir Med 2007;101:399–410.
9. Robinson JA, Crawford G. Identifying palliative care patients with symptoms of depression: an algorithm. Palliat Med 2005;19:278–87.
10. Lilly CM, DeMeo DL, Sonna LA, et al. An intensive communication intervention for the critically ill. Am J Med 2000;109:469–75.
11. Lilly CM, Sonna LA, Haley KJ, et al. Intensive communication: four-year follow-up from a clinical practice study. Crit Care Med 2003;31:S394–9.
12. Linyear AS, Tartaglia A. Family communication coordination: a program to increase organ donation. J Transpl Coord 1999;9:165–74.
13. Jurkevich GJ, Pierce B, Panamen L, et al. Giving bad news: the family perspective. J Trauma 2000;48:865–73.
14. Barber v Superior Court, 147 Cal App3d 1006, 195 Rptr 484 Cal App 2d Dist 1983.
15. Bartling v Superior Court, 163 Cal App3d 186, 209 Cal Rptr 220 1984.
16. Boiuvia v Superior Court, 179 Cal App3d 1127, 225 Cal Rptr 297 1986.
17. Wons v Public Health Trust of Dade County, 500 So2d 679 (Fla App3rd Dist 1987).
18. Medical futility in end-of-life care: report of the Council on Ethical and Judicial Affairs. JAMA 1999;281:937–41.
19. Lamont EB, Christakis NA. Prognostication in advanced disease. In: Berger AM, Portnoy RK, Weissman DE, editors. Principles and practice of palliative care and supportive oncology. 2nd edition. Philadelphia: Lippincott, Williams, and Wilkins; 2002. p. 607–14.
20. Anderson F, Downing GM, Hill J. Palliative performance scale (PPS): a new tool. J Palliat Care 1996;12(1):5–11.
21. Morita T, Tsunoda J, Inoue S, et al. Validity of the palliative performance scale from a survival perspective. J Pain Symptom Manage 1999;18(1):2–3.
22. Virik K, Glare P. Validation of the palliative performance scale for inpatients admitted to a palliative care unit in Sydney, Australia. J Pain Symptom Manage 2002;23(6):455–7.
23. Beauchamp TL, Childress JF. Principles of biomedical ethics. 4th edition. New York: Oxford University Press; 1994. p. 206–11.

24. Muller-Busch H, et al. Sedation in palliative care? A critical analysis of 7 years experience. BMC Palliat Care 2003;2(1):2.
25. Sykes N, Thorns A. Sedative use in the last week of life and the implications for end-of-life decision making. Arch Intern Med 2003;163(2):341–4.
26. von Gunten C and Weissman DE. Fast Facts and Concepts #34: Symptom Control for Ventilator Withdrawal in the Dying Patient; February, 2001. End-of-Life Physician Education Resource Center www.eperc.mcw.edu.
27. Hofmann B, Haheim LL, SÆreide JA. Ethics of palliative surgery in patients with cancer. British Journal of Surgery 2005;92:802–9.
28. Wagman LD (ed). Palliative Surgical Oncology. Surg Oncol Clin N Am 2004;13:401–554.

Subjective Idiopathic Tinnitus and Palliative Care: A Plan for Diagnosis and Treatment

Abraham Shulman, MD, FACS[a,b,]*, Barbara Goldstein, PhD[a,b]

KEYWORDS

- Tinnitology • Clinical types of tinnitus • Tinnitus relief
- Palliation • Tinnitogenesis • Receptor-targeted therapy
- Cognitive-based therapy

The symptom of tinnitus, an aberrant auditory sensory perception, can be a horribly annoying problem for those who are sufferers and a frustrating problem for the physicians, audiologists, and others who are challenged to help these patients find relief from the sounds they are hearing in their head or ears. To some extent, tinnitus is pervasive; reportedly, 12 million people in the United States are troubled by tinnitus.[1] In fact, tinnitus so commonly accompanies presbycusis, the hearing loss that occurs with aging, that many people think tinnitus is just "to be expected as part of growing older."

In this article, the term *tinnitus* refers to subjective idiopathic tinnitus of the severe disabling type (SIT), a neurotologic disorder of the cochleovestibular system, which is acute or chronic in its clinical course, with interference in the life style of the patient.[2]

Despite attempts over many years to identify an underlying cause of tinnitus and its site of lesion and to elucidate the pathophysiology that would explain why tinnitus occurs, tinnitus remains a disorder that must be categorized as idiopathic. Even though the biologic substrate for tinnitus is not well defined and there is no medical or surgical treatment reliably known to eradicate the symptom completely once it has become manifest, patients who have tinnitus can be helped by those doctors and other professionals who have the empathy, inclination, and expertise to offer treatments that can in many ways ameliorate the anguish of patients who have tinnitus.

[a] State University of New York, Downstate, 450 Clarkson Avenue, Box 1239, Brooklyn, NY, USA
[b] Martha Entenmann Tinnitus Research Center, Inc., USA
* Corresponding author. State University of New York, Downstate, 450 Clarkson Avenue, Box 1239, Brooklyn, NY.
E-mail address: metrc@inch.com (A. Shulman).

Otolaryngol Clin N Am 42 (2009) 15–37
doi:10.1016/j.otc.2008.09.012
0030-6665/08/$ – see front matter © 2009 Elsevier Inc. All rights reserved.

At the Tinnitus Clinic of the Department of Otolaryngology, State University of New York, Downstate, and at the Martha Entenmann Tinnitus Research Center, Inc., since 1979, experience has been amassed with 10,000 patients who have SIT. Although the authors and their colleagues have varying levels of success in offering treatment for their patients, the basic tenet of their program is the age-old adage, "first, do no harm." Thus, in a sense, although the authors accept the fact that eradication of the symptom of tinnitus may not be an achievable goal for many patients who come to them seeking help, they do aim to provide palliation.

Palliation has been defined as treatment given to relieve symptoms.[3] Palliation also implies a treatment consisting of disguising or concealing a disease. Palliative medicine is oriented to relief of the symptom rather than the underlying causal pathologic condition, with the intention of improving the quality of life (QOL) for the patient. Palliation medicine for otolaryngology has been limited and has focused primarily on symptoms associated with malignant disease of the head and neck (eg, pain control, relief and maintenance of function of the food and air passageways, hospice care).

A palliative approach for the patient who has SIT can be considered in terms of tinnitus relief achieved with combined treatment protocols, highlighted by medication and instrumentation, to achieve and maintain a QOL consistent with the goals of the individual patient (ie, maintenance of auditory function and communication abilities, physical integrity of the cochleovestibular system and normal brain function, normal behavioral psychologic responses in the presence of tinnitus, adequate sleep, participation in social activities).

Palliation for SIT combines a holistic, compassionate, symptomatic, and interdisciplinary approach to achieve at least a modicum of relief and is based on the application of varying regimens that have been developed, with information coming from advances in the understanding of auditory, brain, neural pathway, and psychodynamic functions.

CONCEPTS AND PROTOCOLS FOR TINNITUS DIAGNOSIS AND TREATMENT

The following concepts of palliative medicine from the literature, when integrated with those that have evolved from the authors' clinical experiences with SIT protocols of diagnosis and treatment, are resulting in increasing success in achieving relief for the patient who has SIT.

PRINCIPLES OF PALLIATIVE CARE FOR SUBJECTIVE IDIOPATHIC TINNITUS OF THE SEVERE DISABLING TYPE

The evolution of the discipline of palliation medicine is well established in the twenty-first century and has witnessed the inclusion of nonmalignant disease, beyond quality-of-life (QOL) issues and hospice care for malignant disease, by application of clinical experiences for pain relief in nonmalignant conditions; in patients who have chronic diseases, symptoms, or injury; and in therapies directed to QOL issues.[4]

The statement of principles developed by the Task Force on Surgical Palliative Care and the Committee on Ethics of the American College of Surgeons (ACS) in 2005 reflects this evolution to a broad range of patients receiving surgical care.[5]

The following principles of palliative care for subjective SIT are recommended, reflecting modification and clinical application of the principles of palliative care proposed by the ACS:[5]

1. Respect the dignity and autonomy of patients who have tinnitus, patients' surrogates, and caregivers.

2. Respect and honor the right of the competent patient or surrogate to choose among treatments, including those that may or may not provide tinnitus relief.
3. Communicate effectively and empathetically with patients, their families, and caregivers.
4. Identify the primary goals of care from the patient's perspective, and address how the professional attempting tinnitus relief can achieve the patient's objectives and present the realities and limitations of what is and is not known about tinnitus.
5. Do the best one can to achieve tinnitus relief, establish the medical significance of the tinnitus, and differentiate in treatment recommendations among the components of all sensations (ie, sensation, affect behavioral response to the sensation, psychomotor response to the sensation).
6. Recognize, assess, discuss, and offer access to services of neurology, psychology or psychiatry, social issues, tinnitus patient support groups, and national and international tinnitus organizations.
7. Provide access to therapeutic support when such support can realistically be expected to improve the QOL as perceived by the patient.
8. Recognize the physician's responsibility to discourage treatments that are unlikely to achieve the patient's goals.
9. Arrange for continuity of care by the patient's primary or specialist physician or audiologist, alleviating the sense of abandonment that patients may feel when "curative" therapies are not available. Do not tell a patient, "You have to live with it."
10. Maintain a collegial and supportive attitude toward others entrusted with the care of the patient.

PALLIATION MEDICINE AND TINNITUS: A BIOPHYSIOLOGIC MODEL

The landmark neuroscience contributions of Eric Kandel[6] to the understanding of mind and memory are considered to provide, in part, a biophysiologic model to explain the symptomatic relief with palliative medicine, particularly with combined therapies of counseling and drug therapy for control of anxiety and medication, both of which are significant for the patient who has SIT. Specifically, it has been demonstrated that "talk" therapy and listening to the patient involve the brain pathways within the frontal lobes that are involved primarily in cognitive processing (ie, "thinking.") Neural processing is primarily "top down." Fluorodeoxyglucose (FDG) positron emission tomography (PET) brain nuclear medicine imaging has demonstrated an increase in activity in the caudate nucleus in patients who have obsessive-compulsive disorder.[7]

Drug therapy with selective serotonin receptor inhibitors (SSRIs) has been identified to work primarily in subcortical "nonthinking" brain regions (ie, neural processing is primarily "bottom up.") For SIT, this rationale is hypothesized to provide, in part, an explanation for the relief from SIT reported with combined therapies directed to the sensory and affect components of the SIT—specifically, the ultimate influence on the processes involved in the establishment of paradoxical auditory memory, the initial process in transformation of an aberrant auditory sensory stimulus (SIT) to an affect behavioral response (ie, the final common pathway for tinnitus).[8,9] The differences in relief for SIT are based on the underlying molecular genetics involved in sensory, affect, and cognitive processing, which reflect the individuality of each patient who has SIT and the heterogeneity of tinnitus in general and SIT in particular.

QUALITY OF LIFE

QOL issues for a particular symptom or disease are individual and subjective for each patient. Reports of QOL in patients who have tinnitus should always differentiate between SIT and other clinical types of tinnitus (CTTs).[10–12]

QOL determinants for SIT have been individual in the authors' clinical medical audiologic neurotology experience with SIT in excess of 10,000 patients since 1979, originating in the Tinnitus Clinic of the Department of Otolaryngology, State University of New York, Downstate, and ongoing at the Martha Entenmann Tinnitus Research Center, Inc. The authors' experience has been marked by the heterogeneity and diversity of influences and end points for SIT QOL issues, including physical, psychologic, and social components. For SIT, QOL issues are highlighted by interference in sleep, concentration, communication, performance at work, and interference in social activities with family and friends, with accompanying or resultant anxiety or depression and interference in speech expression and memory. Most important in evaluating reports of QOL issues and tinnitus is the clinical diagnosis of the type of tinnitus. In this article, tinnitus refers to subjective SIT.[10]

In the authors' experience, a team approach of the primary physician and otology-neurotology, audiology, and neuropsychology or psychiatry specialists with a resultant stable personality increases the efficacy of modality(ies) of therapy attempting relief from SIT and the resultant QOL for the patient who has SIT.

Significant determinants have been identified to influence the clinical course of the SIT, the efficacy of therapies attempting tinnitus relief, and the resultant QOL of the patient who has SIT. Included are the following:[2]

- Affect/behavioral response to the presence of SIT: the antecedent or associated behavioral affect response of anxiety and depression to the presence of the SIT is the most significant determinant for the QOL in most patients who have SIT.
- Parameters of tinnitus identification of quality of tone and/or noise, intensity, location, masking effect(s), and duration: intensity is the most frequent complaint influencing the QOL (ie, the higher the intensity, the greater is the report of interference in QOL). The next most frequent complaint has been duration (ie, the longer the duration, the greater is the report of interference in QOL). Individual, occasional, and less frequent has been the report of influence of the quality of the SIT (single or multiple, tone or noise, and location) on SIT QOL. Sociodemographic factors associated with SIT include age, stress, and noise exposure; antecedent neuropsychiatric disease (eg, anxiety; depression; posttraumatic stress disorder [PTSD]; traumatic brain injury [TBI]; metabolic disease of sugar, thyroid, or hyperlipidemia; cardiovascular disease); identification, treatment, or control of hypertension or arrhythmias; and neuropsychiatric disease (eg, anxiety, depression, cerebrovascular or neurodegenerative central system [CNS] disease). Age alone has not been a significant factor for SIT except when associated with neuropsychiatric disease and neurodegenerative CNS disease.
- Neurotologic-associated conditions: Neurotologic conditions associated with SIT, as identified by the patient's history, physical examination and cochleovestibular testing, have been identified and are known to influence the clinical course of the SIT adversely. When not identified and controlled, such conditions have been reported to influence adversely the QOL of the patient who has SIT. Included are the presence of hyperacusis, sensorineural hearing loss, fluctuation in aeration of the middle ears, secondary endolymphatic hydrops (SEH), noise exposure, and stress.[10,13]

Erlandsson and Hallberg[14] reported on the QOL and its association with tinnitus-related factors (psychologic, psychosomatic, and audiologic) based on a sample of 122 patients who attended a hearing clinic for distress as a result of tinnitus. Six of 13 variables included in the model proved to be significant regressors and to explain 65% of the variance. The 6 predictor variables were as follows:

1. Impaired concentration
2. Feeling depressed
3. Perceived negative attitudes
4. Hypersensitivity to sounds
5. Average hearing level (best ear)
6. Tinnitus duration (the shorter the duration of tinnitus, the more negative was the impact on QOL)

The three most significant predictors were directly related to perceived psychologic distress and explained most of the variance in QOL in the patients who had tinnitus and were included in this study. An unexpected finding was that fluctuations in tinnitus, vertigo, headache, or perceived social support did not prove to belong to the significant regressors.[15]

A recent report highlights the significance of the impact of tinnitus on QOL in older patients who have tinnitus.[15] In a population-based study, in self-reported data using the Medical Outcomes Study Short Form Health Survey (SF-36) from 2800 subjects who were aged 53 to 97 years, with 669 subjects having a mild, moderate, or severe level of tinnitus, the most significant negative effects of tinnitus showed up in the domains of physical pain and stress, as opposed to the mental and emotional domains. When looking at the SF-36 data, mean scores for all eight domains (physical functioning, role-physical, bodily pain, general hearing perceptions, vitality, social functioning, role-emotional, and mental health index) worsened with the severity of the subject's tinnitus, as did mean scores for the two summary indexes (Physical Summary and Mental Component Summary). A significant ($P<.05$) linear trend was observed for the role-physical, bodily pain, vitality, and Physical Component Summary index. Almost 25% of the population had tinnitus, with 9.4% reporting moderate to severe tinnitus. The researchers concluded that "quality of life is diminished in participants with tinnitus, and the effect increases with severity."[15]

Reports of QOL in patients who have tinnitus should always differentiate between SIT and other CTTs.[10–12]

TINNITOLOGY

Tinnitology is a new distinct discipline that has been identified, defined, and developed since 1991.[16] It has become a multidiscipline of professionals dedicated to the study of tinnitus and to the translation and integration of clinical otology with the behavioral and basic sciences for tinnitus diagnosis and treatment. Specifically, basic scientists, clinicians, and audiologists are attempting to understand how an aberrant auditory sensation (ie, tinnitus) is transformed into an affect behavioral response. Tinnitology is evolving as an integrated multidiscipline of basic science, auditory science, neuroscience, and clinical medicine. Modalities of treatment recommended at this time are resulting in tinnitus relief (ie, palliation) in an increasing number of cases.

DEFINITIONS AND CLASSIFICATION

Definitions of "tinnitus" are dynamic, reflecting what is and is not known of auditory science, sensory biophysiology, the cochleovestibular system (peripheral and central), the brain (structure and function), and human behavior. Originally the definition focused on its subjective nature and was defined as the perception of an aberrant auditory stimulus unrelated to an external source of sound.[17]

In 1992, tinnitus was defined as a sensory disorder of auditory perception reflecting an aberrant auditory signal produced by interference in the excitatory or inhibitory process(es) involved in neurotransmission. This definition reflected the integration of clinical efforts of observation with neuroscience and nuclear medicine to identify underlying mechanisms of tinnitus and to establish the medical significance of tinnitus.

In 2006, tinnitus was defined as a clinical conscious awareness, varying in degree of consolidation, of an aberrant auditory paradoxical memory originating in response to an interference in the homeostasis between dyssynchrony and synchrony within the synaptic circuitry of the neural substrates involved, and thus interfering in the precision, specificity, and complexity involved in synaptic transmission for normal neuronal and interneuronal function.[9]

A tinnitus classification system has been recommended differentiating between an otologic and neurotologic clinical site of lesion.[10–12] The otologic classification is based on the integration of the clinical history and otologic physical examination. The neurotologic examination is based on extrapolation of correlates of electrophysiologic testing of the cochlear vestibular system, peripheral or central in location. The neurotologic or otologic classification primarily provides a basis for the diagnosis of SIT and the selection of a suitable system method for tinnitus treatment and tinnitus control. It offers a method for standardizing the reporting of SIT data for its diagnosis and treatment.

Classification based on epidemiology is further recommended to differentiate between clinical and subclinical tinnitus and auditory and nonauditory tinnitus (ie, whether the auditory system is the primary site of origin of the lesion of the tinnitus complaint [auditory tinnitus] or whether it is secondarily involved [nonauditory tinnitus]).[10–12,18] Other system(s) may use the auditory system to express the dysfunction. Clinically manifest tinnitus is an auditory threshold perception that the patient is experiencing. Subclinical tinnitus refers to the tinnitus as an abnormal subthreshold auditory sensation. Tinnitus may be subclinical in nature and become clinically manifest with a "trigger" event. Such an event may be that of noise exposure or inflammation, for example.

PRINCIPLES OF CLINICAL TINNITOLOGY

The following principles of tinnitology reflect the realities of the authors' experiences for tinnitus diagnosis and treatment at this time. To be informed and to share information with the patient are principles of palliative medicine.

Principles have evolved from attempts at establishing accuracy for the clinical diagnosis of tinnitus and for attempting tinnitus relief in 2007 through 2008, which have been called "principles of tinnitology" and include the following:[19]

1. There is no cure for tinnitus at this time.[10]
2. Treatment efficacy is based on the accuracy of the tinnitus diagnosis.[10]
3. Not all tinnitus is the same. It is necessary to differentiate tinnitus in patients with the symptoms of SIT from tinnitus that is occasional or tinnitus that is present and not disabling.[10–12]
4. Tinnitus is not a unitary symptom. There are different CTTs and clinical subtypes of tinnitus.[18]
5. The masking of tinnitus is reflected in different types of masking.[20]

6. Tinnitus is reflected in its clinical course as a chronic, multifactorial, heterogeneous complaint.[10]
7. Components of tinnitus have been identified based on a clinical translation of basic sensory physiology for tinnitus diagnosis and treatment (ie, sensory, affect, psychomotor).[21]
8. Factors have been identified that influence the clinical course of the SIT. When treated, the result is significant tinnitus relief.[2]
9. Noise is a significant etiology influencing the clinical course of the tinnitus. Increasing noise exposure results in an increase in the intensity of tinnitus.[10]
10. Stress exacerbates the intensity of tinnitus. A stress diathesis model for tinnitus has been hypothesized.[8,22,23]
11. Tinnitus has medical significance for each patient who has tinnitus, which requires an attempt to be established.[24]
12. Management realities: although there is no cure for tinnitus at this time, there are systems available for attempting tinnitus relief, which are highlighted by medication and instrumentation.[10,19,25,26]
13. Treatment recommendations are based on a dilemma that has and does exist for the symptoms of tinnitus and aberrant auditory phenomena unrelated to an external source of sound. Specifically, the question is how a sensory phenomenon becomes transposed or translated to one of affect or how the reverse can take place.[8,27]
14. A final common pathway in the brain has been hypothesized for all CTTs, with the initial process(es) being the establishment of a paradoxical auditory memory for the aberrant auditory stimulus (**Fig. 1**). "The chief function is the transition of a dyssynchronous auditory sensory signal to affective behavioral response. It is hypothesized that for all sensory systems, the sensory and affect components are linked by memory."[8]

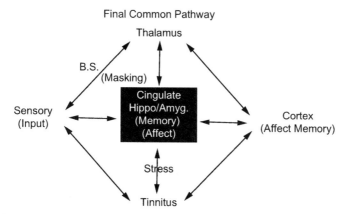

Fig. 1. Final common pathway for tinnitus, 1995. A reciprocal, innervating, interneuronal network transforms a sensory aberrant stimulus, tinnitus, to one of affect and emotion. The factor of stress and the biophysiologic processes involved modulate the severity of the tinnitus. Amyg, amygdala; B.S., brain stem; Hippo, hippocampus. (*From* Shulman A. A final common pathway for tinnitus: the medial temporal lobe system. Int Tinnitus J 1995;1:119; with permission.)

15. The key to efficacy for tinnitus treatment depends on the accuracy of the diagnosis for tinnitus. The completion of a medical audiologic tinnitus patient protocol (MATPP) (**Fig. 2**), with examination of the cochleovestibular system (ear and brain), improves the accuracy of the SIT diagnosis and efficacy of modality(ies) recommended for attempting tinnitus relief.[2,28]

16. A biochemical marker, the γ-aminobutyric acid-A receptor (GABA-AR) has been identified for a predominantly central type of tinnitus. Its clinical application is a therapy targeting the GABA-AR, which is resulting in long-term tinnitus relief.[29]

17. An electrophysiologic correlate has been identified for a predominantly central type of tinnitus[30]

18. Receptor-targeted therapy (RTT) directed to the GABA-AR called RTT-GABA has resulted in the clinical treatment application for a patient who has the predominantly central type of SIT.[31]

19. Tinnitus is not a phantom phenomenon. Electrodiagnostic, physiologic, and biochemical alterations in neural substrates have been identified, which are significant for different CTTs.[8,29,31]

20. The ultrahigh audiometric response can be used for the identification of patients who have SIT and may benefit from acoustic stimulation using ultrahigh-frequency stimulation.[32,33]

PRINCIPLES OF SENSORY PHYSIOLOGY

The basic tenet of sensory physiology that there are different clinical components for any sensation has been clinically applied for the patient who has SIT. The components are sensory, affect, and psychomotor.[21] For tinnitus the sensory component is the tinnitus symptom itself, the affect component is the behavioral response of the patient who has tinnitus to the presence of the tinnitus, and the psychomotor component is the somatomotor response to the behavioral component of the tinnitus.[19]

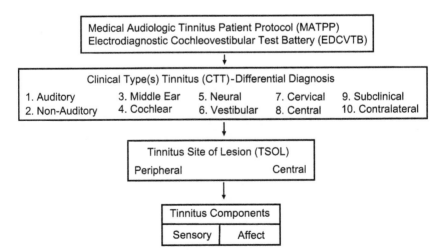

Fig. 2. MATPP: diagnosis and treatment. (*From* Shulman A. Medical audiologic tinnitus patient protocol. In: Shulman A, et al, editors. Tinnitus diagnosis/treatment. Forest Hills (NY): Martha Entenmann Tinnitus Research Foundation, Inc. p. 109; with permission.)

Tinnitus is an aberrant auditory sensation. Recommendations for tinnitus relief should specify and differentiate among the components of the aberrant auditory sensation (ie, tinnitus).

In general, for the SIT sensory component, a combination of instrumentation and medication is advised. For the affect component focusing predominantly on anxiety and depression, appropriate anxiolytic and antidepressant medications are recommended. Fear is a significant factor in new patients who have SIT, and appropriate psychiatric medication or psychotherapy is recommended. To be considered is that a significant number of patients, particularly in the geriatric age population, have associated complaints of interference in memory and cognition. Appropriate neurodegenerative drugs or memory enhancers are recommended.

TINNITOGENESIS

Tinnitogenesis is a seizure type activity, cortical-subcortical in location, with a resultant aberrant auditory perception.[34] It is an epileptiform auditory phenomenon. It is hypothesized that a disruption in calcium homeostasis reflective of glutamate neurotoxicity results in hyperexcitability in the underlying neural substrate of epileptiform characteristics. This finding has provided a rationale for the innovative recommendation of antiepileptic agents in an attempt to achieve tinnitus relief in appropriate patients who have SIT.

MEDICAL SIGNIFICANCE OF TINNITUS

The medical significance of tinnitus is considered to be the spectrum of clinical manifestations reflecting interference in function of the cochleovestibular system or brain, with sensory, affect, and psychomotor components.[2,24] The sensory component is considered to be the tinnitus sound and quality. The affect component is the patient's behavioral response to the tinnitus. The psychomotor component is a somatomotor response to the behavioral component of tinnitus.

The otologic and neurotologic etiologies associated with the medical significance of tinnitus have been found to be highlighted by associations with inflammatory disease of the middle ear or mastoid, Ménière's disease, acoustic tumor, sensorineural hearing loss, and autoimmune inner ear disease.

TINNITUS THEORIES: DIAGNOSIS AND TREATMENT APPLICATIONS

Hypotheses of mechanisms of tinnitus in the past included changes in temporal firing patterns of neuronal activity,[35,36] "cross-talk" among eighth nerve fibers,[37] analogy to pain perception,[38] damage to the temporal dysfunction of the inner or outer hair cells,[39–42] partial damage to interruption of the eighth nerve,[43] damage to the efferent system,[44,45] imbalanced activity in eighth nerve resulting in tinnitus,[46] and the recent tinnitus dyssynchrony/synchrony theory (**Fig. 3**) to differentiate between the dyssynchronous signal that is hypothesized to be tinnitus and the synchrony of neuronal activity at the brain cortex that is the function of the perception and conscious awareness of tinnitus (see **Fig. 2**).[9]

DIAGNOSIS: CLINICAL ATTEMPT AT OBJECTIFICATION OF TINNITUS—MEDICAL AUDIOLOGIC TINNITUS PATIENT PROTOCOL

Basic principles of neurotology have been followed since 1975 for tinnitus diagnosis and treatment,[28] which are limited by current understanding of the cochleovestibular system and brain function. Protocols recommended for sensorineural hearing loss,

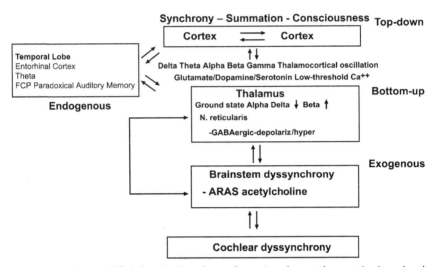

Fig. 3. Integrated model for the tinnitus dyssynchrony/synchrony theory: tinnitus development, propagation, brain function, final common pathway (FCP) for tinnitus. It is hypothesized that a homeostasis of neuroanatomic substrates and neurotransmitters regulates dyssynchrony and synchrony for sensory input received at the brain cortex from the peripheral nervous system or central nervous system (CNS). Rhythmic oscillations modulated by the thalamus are recorded at the cortex and reflect brain function (ie, delta, theta, alpha, beta, gamma). The sensory information ascends by way of the ascending reticular activating system (ARAS) to the thalamus, part of an exogenous system of the CNS for receipt of sensory information arising from the environment or the peripheral nervous system or central CNS. Hyperpolarization and depolarization of GABA-influenced thalamic neuron activity results in thalamocortical oscillations that displace a theoretic ground state of brain activity from the alpha-rhythm down to a theta- or delta-rhythm or up to a beta-rhythm. Input from the thalamus to the temporal lobe and the entorhinal cortex, an endogenous system of the CNS, is hypothesized to result in the establishment of a "memory" for the sensory stimulus, which has a reciprocal influence on the thalamus. The summation of synchronous neural discharges from multiple neural ensembles of neurons at the cortex results in a gamma-rhythm associated with a conscious awareness of the sensory stimulus. Synchronized neural activity in multiple neuronal ensembles is hypothesized to be the basis of perception and consciousness. (*From* Shulman A, Goldstein B. Tinnitus dyssynchrony/synchrony theory: a translational concept for tinnitus diagnosis and treatment. Int Tinnitus J 2006;12:320; with permission.)

vertigo, and ear blockage were modified initially for tinnitus. The clinical goals have been to establish the accuracy of a diagnosis of tinnitus, objectify a subjective aberrant sensory complaint, identify factors influencing the clinical course of the tinnitus, establish its medical significance, and attempt tinnitus relief. Clinicians have been impressed by the heterogeneity of the complaint; the predominance in the clinical complaint of the demonstration of the emotional and behavioral responses of the patient to the presence of the tinnitus; and the influence of noise, exposure, and stress on the clinical course of the tinnitus complaint. The dilemma presented to the basic scientist and clinician was identified as how to explain the transposition of a sensory complaint to one of affect, and how the affect and emotional states of the patient influenced the sensory complaint. Attempts to find the answer to this question are not new. Descartes attempted to answer this question in his own time.[27]

In general, in the authors' experience, the population that has SIT is vulnerable, highlighted by the subjective nature of the complaint and limitations of the medical audiologic professionals in what is and is not known in auditory science about an aberrant auditory sensory complaint (ie, SIT), brain function, behavior, and an understanding of the transformation of a sensory complaint to one of affect. These limitations result in frustration for patients and professionals attempting to establish an accurate diagnosis for SIT (and its relief), which is highlighted by increasing anxiety and depression for the patient and interference in that individual's QOL. Prognostication is a frequent question from the patient who has SIT, and, in the authors' experience, it cannot be predicted. Noise exposure and stress are two factors that are accompanied by the onset and increase in intensity of SIT.

The authors' approach to find answers to this complicated question has recognized the need to consider the totality of the cochleovestibular system (peripheral and central) and brain function. Initially, starting in 1975, a clinical approach for the evaluation of the patient who had tinnitus followed a protocol called the MATPP, which included testing of the totality of the cochleovestibular system (peripheral and central), central speech testing when appropriate, and auditory evoked response short-latency evoked response testing (see **Fig. 3**).[28]

The MATPP is recommended for all patients who have tinnitus of a severe disabling type. It includes the following:

A. History
B. General medical evaluation
C. Neurotologic examination
D. Cochlear vestibular evaluation
E. Tinnitus evaluation: to include testing for the Feldmann masking curves and loudness discomfort levels

The MATPP is a multidisciplinary team approach advised for the medical and audiologic evaluation of SIT, which is a neurotologic complaint. Specialists include those in the areas of otology, audiology, family medicine, internal medicine, neurology, psychiatry, and psychology. The neurotologic evaluation is a team approach of audiology and medicine having as its goal the identification of CTTs; identification and treatment of factor(s) influencing the clinical course of SIT; and determination of the medical significance of tinnitus with respect to the general health of the patient and its audiologic significance, particularly with respect to hearing function and communication abilities of the patient and brain function.

The masking curves of Feldmann, which have been shown to be individual for each patient who has tinnitus, provide a basis for the identification of clinical types of SIT, the suitability of masking for the patient who has tinnitus, and the ear to be selected for a masker.[20] When used alone or in combination with a hearing aid, the reduction of the intensity of tinnitus is reported by the patient during its use and by residual inhibition in a postmasking stimulation (partial or total).

Since 1977, the MATPP has emphasized the ear more than the brain. The patient's clinical history has been crucial for diagnosis and has included identification of the parameters of tinnitus identification (ie, quality, location, intensity, masking, rebound). An attempt was made to associate the report of tinnitus with complaint(s) of hearing loss, vertigo, ear blockage, stress, and central nervous system (CNS) symptoms. Factors were identified that were known to contribute to the clinical course of the tinnitus. Such systemic factors were highlighted by cardiovascular (ie, hypertension, cardiac arrhythmias), metabolic (ie, sugar, hyperlipidemias), endocrine (ie, glucose, thyroid), and CNS (ie, cerebrovascular disease, mild cognitive impairment) abnormalities.

Additional factors of noise exposure, stress, anxiety, and depression have all been recognized to be associated with increasing intensity of tinnitus.

What is needed for the twenty-first century are increasing methods to objectify the tinnitus clinically and to consider the ear and brain to be equally significant for the diagnosis and treatment of tinnitus. The clinical history should include what has been described, with additional emphasis on the CNS (ie, taste, smell, memory, speech expression, cognition, consciousness) and the mind. The eliciting of the clinical history as described continues to be significant in establishing the diagnosis of tinnitus. A family history of hearing loss, stress, emotion, anxiety, and depression is equally significant. The electrodiagnostic cochleovestibular evaluation gained significance with the addition of two tests: quantitative electroencephalography (QEEG)[30] and craniocorpography (CCG).[47,48] QEEG is a multimetric spectral analysis of the raw electroencephalography. CCG is a vestibular test system that also provides information about the psychomotor component of the tinnitus. The introduction of QEEG and CCG has provided electrophysiologic measures for tinnitus and balance diagnoses reflecting brain function in the patient who has tinnitus. Nuclear medicine imaging (MRI) of the brain for structure and single photon emission computed tomography (SPECT), positron emission tomography (PET), and CT-PET for function and the coregistration of data provide a metabolic measure of brain activity in multiple neural substrates in the patient who has SIT. Both provide electrophysiologic and metabolic measures of activity in the brain that have been translated for clinical application in the patient who has SIT for understanding underlying mechanisms of tinnitus production, increased accuracy of tinnitus diagnosis, and a monitoring technique to evaluate objectively the efficacy of modalities of treatment recommended for attempting tinnitus relief.[8,28,30,34,49–54]

The complaint of hyperacusis must be identified for each patient who has tinnitus.[55] A loudness discomfort level test is routinely performed. Different clinical types of hyperacusis have been described.

The MATPP has provided a basis for clinically attempting to objectify the subjective complaint of tinnitus. This led to the identification of different CTTs by the extrapolation of the cochleovestibular test findings as electrophysiologic correlates of cochleovestibular function and dysfunction and their integration with the clinical history and neurotologic physical examination for accurate diagnosis of tinnitus. The hypothesis that tinnitus could have its origin in the central or peripheral cochleovestibular system was clinically considered to be supported by the cochleovestibular test findings highlighted by the auditory brainstem response (ABR) results.[56,57]

SEVERE IDIOPATHIC TINNITUS CLINICAL HISTORY AND PALLIATIVE MEDICINE

Principles of palliative medicine in general and chronic complaints highlighted by pain management specifically have found application for chronic SIT, which is persistent or recurrent in excess of 6 to 12 months. Analogies between pain and tinnitus have been proposed. Tinnitus can be considered to be pain of the auditory system (Juergen Tonndorf, MD, PhD, personal communication, 1989).

A cardinal principle of palliative medicine followed in the MATPP, in an attempt to provide relief of SIT, is the importance of listening and allowing adequate time for obtaining a complete medical neurotologic and audiologic history of the SIT complaint. Highlights include the following:

- Identify the parameters of identification of SIT at the time of consultation and time of onset.

- Establish metrics for identification of intensity and annoyance at the time of onset compared with that at consultation and follow-up visits (ie, to appreciate and identify the clinical course of SIT).
- Attempt a complete review of systems, stressing the association of SIT with the following:
  1. Cochleovestibular complaints highlighted by hearing loss, vertigo, ear blockage, and hyperacusis
  2. Ear, nose, and throat (ENT) complaints of otalgia (eg, dysfunction, hearing loss, inflammatory ear or nose sinus disease during childhood or as an adult)
  3. CNS complaint(s) reflective of the cranial nerves 1 through 12, highlighted by vision, smell, headache, cognition, speech expression, memory, motor function, and gait
  4. Metabolic disorders (eg, disorders of sugar, thyroid, and lipids)
  5. Cardiovascular disorders (eg, hypertension, atrial fibrillation, coronary atherosclerosis)
  6. Skeletal-muscular disorders (eg, cervical osteoarthritis)
  7. Menses (present or absent, replacement hormonal therapy)
  8. Pain (anatomic location, intensity, timing, medication, quality and what [if any] association with the reported SIT)
- Establish a noise and stress profile and their correlation to the clinical course of the patient who has SIT.
- Obtain a psychiatric history of patient with a focus on anxiety, depression, and medications received (with a positive or negative effect) for SIT.
- Obtain list of medications dispensed by a pharmacy to the patient for any and all complaint(s) in the year before consultation.
- Obtain prior test results (eg, audiometric or vestibular testing, brain or ear imaging).
- Obtain a list of treatment modalities attempted for relief of SIT and results (self-prescribed).
- Obtain a list of stimulants used by the patient (eg, coffee, alcohol, smoking).
- Obtain a family history focusing on disorders of the immune system, allergy, hearing loss, diabetes mellitus, epilepsy, or other illnesses in the family.

CLINICAL TYPES OF TINNITUS

CTTs are identified by means of completion by the patient of a MATPP.[10–13,28,57] The consideration of CTTs is not new.[58]

CTTs (eg, auditory or nonauditory, clinical or subclinical) reflect the degree of ability or inability of a dyssynchronous signal to become synchronous and to establish itself as a conscious percept of memory. The establishment of and consolidation of a paradoxical auditory memory for an aberrant auditory signal reflects itself clinically in the degree of severity of tinnitus.[8–13,28,29]

TINNITUS IS NOT A PHANTOM PHENOMENON

Tinnitus has been characterized as an auditory phantom disorder.[59,60] In the past, the term *phantom* has been applied when no neural substrate or underlying processes involved in sensory coding are known. Tinnitus is considered to reflect the basic problem in sensory physiology (ie, sensory coding). "True code" has been defined as a parameter of the signal that actually carries behaviorally useful information.[61]

Tinnitus is not a "phantom" but an active physical process or phenomenon occurring in multiple neural substrates in response to a peripheral or central stimulus identifiable in electrophysiologic recordings (cortical and subcortical and metabolic activated neural substrates) reflecting a synchrony/desynchrony in homeostatic mechanisms involved in the maintenance of "normal" individual brain function. The identification of neural substrates in the brain with nuclear medicine imaging and QEEG electrophysiologic patterns of response at the cortex supports the recommendation that tinnitus is not to be considered a phantom phenomenon.[8,30,49–54]

TREATMENT
General

Treatment of a symptom implies identification of its etiology and understanding of the known underlying pathophysiologic mechanisms involved, with the expectation of a cure.[2,25,26] Modalities of therapy attempting tinnitus relief at this time (eg, medication, surgery, instrumentation) are achieving palliation (ie, relief of the symptoms). They are based on clinical translation of theories of underlying mechanism(s) of tinnitus production, principles of the basic science of sensory physiology, identification and treatment of factor(s) influencing the clinical course of the SIT, and treatment providing neuroprotection.[2,25,26,61–74]

Treatment strategies attempting tinnitus relief since 1995 have been called tinnitus-targeted therapy (TTT), which has tinnitus relief (ie, palliation) as its goal. TTT is an SIT treatment protocol that includes the combination of medication or instrumentation targeting biophysiologic mechanisms hypothesized to underlie the initiation, propagation, and clinical course of the symptoms of different CTTs and the identification and medical treatment of local and systemic disease. Neuropsychiatric disease or complaints require identification and treatment.

In the authors' experience, attempts at tinnitus relief for all CTTs have increased by (1) completion of the MATPP for the identification of the CTT and identification and treatment of factor(s) influencing the clinical course of the tinnitus, (2) follow-up of the realities and guidelines for the principles of tinnitology, and (3) clinical translation of principles of basic sensory physiology for recommendations attempting tinnitus relief.

Tinnitus is a chronic complaint.[10] Two essential elements have been recognized for treatment: the sensory component (the tinnitus itself) and the behavioral response to the sensation.

The authors' overall results for medical tinnitus relief since 2000 are positive in approximately 85% to 90% of patients who have SIT. The recommendation for instrumentation has been reduced as the result of an increase in long-term tinnitus relief with medication. The breakdown for tinnitus relief with medication overall efficacy since 2000 has been 85% (10% with instrumentation using masking, amplification, or external electrical stimulation). The remaining 5% to 10% continue to be problem cases. These patients have been identified clinically as having a primarily central type of SIT existing alone or in combination with other CTTs.

The following is a brief summary of the protocols recommended for attempting tinnitus relief. The reader is referred to appropriate references cited in this article for additional information and details of the recommendations.

MEDICAL TREATMENT
Treatment Sensory Component

Factors that influence the clinical course of tinnitus
Factors influencing the clinical course of the tinnitus, when identified and treated, have been found to result in tinnitus relief.[10,13,19,25] Failure for such identification has been

found to interfere in the efficacy of recommendations of medication or instrumentation attempting tinnitus relief.[2,10]

Secondary endolymphatic hydrops

SEH has been found in patients who have SIT with or without vertigo.[2,10,13,18] Treatment is recommended with diuretic therapy, antihistamines, and diet-elimination stimulants. The incidence of occurrence of SEH is approximately 35% in the authors' series overall. The control of SEH indirectly contributes to tinnitus relief by increasing the efficacy of the recommendation of instrumentation attempting tinnitus relief and stabilization of the sensorineural hearing loss.

Fluctuation in aeration of the middle ear

Fluctuation in aeration of the middle ear may influence tinnitus intensity.[2,10,19] Its identification is attributable to inflammatory or allergic conditions of the nose, paranasal sinuses, and throat in addition to secondary Eustachian tube dysfunction. Treatment with systemic antihistamine or decongestant medication and local treatment, including pneumatoscopy, have resulted in tinnitus relief in approximately 10% to 15% of the authors' patients who have SIT.

Noise control

Adequate noise protection with ear defenders and avoidance of noise are recommended.[2,10] Compliance is critical for any recommendations attempting tinnitus relief.

Metabolic factors of abnormalities in sugar, cholesterol, triglyceride, and thyroid function, alone or in combination, may influence the clinical course of sensorineural hearing loss and SIT. Treatment involves identification and follow-up with an internist to ensure satisfactory control.[2,10,19] Synergy has been questioned between hypertension, hyperlipidemias, and noise exposure, resulting in gradual progressive sensorineural hearing loss.[66]

Patients who have SIT with hypercholesterolemia and triglyceride elevation have also reported tinnitus relief with treatment attempting to improve the oxygen-carrying capacity of blood. Trental, 40 mg, titrated to once a day or a maximum of three times a day is recommended if there are no medical contraindications.[2,10,19]

Cardiovascular factors

Fluctuation in hypertension is, in the authors' experience, the most frequent significant cardiovascular factor involved in the clinical course of SIT. Its identification and control are considered fundamental for any attempt at tinnitus relief. Cardiac arrhythmias, particularly auricular fibrillation with potential consequences for emboli formation, are significant. It is recommended that treatment be directed by an internist.[2,10,19]

Cerebrovascular factors

Cerebrovascular disease, epilepsy, and memory and cognitive disorders, when identified and treated in appropriate patients who have SIT, have been found to be accompanied by relief of SIT. Effective drugs include the vasodilator papaverine for cerebrovascular insufficiency, Plavix in patients who have had a transient ischemic attack(s) or stroke, and antiseizure drugs for epilepsy. For memory and cognition, the neuroprotective drugs Aricept, tacrine, memantine, gabapentin, and Klonopin are recommended. These drugs attempt to improve the status of the underlying neuronal substrate that may be contributing to SIT.[19]

Otosclerosis

Otosclerosis, when identified by integration of the clinical history and tomographic examination of the temporal bones, is considered to be a factor influencing the clinical course of tinnitus. Treatment is recommended starting with a Didronate, 400 mg, once a day for 2 weeks, followed by calcium carbonate with vitamin D for 4 weeks, to be repeated every 3 months[19,67]

Treatment Affect Component-Affective Disorders, Anxiety, and Depression

Affective disorders highlighted by anxiety and depression are significant complaints associated with SIT.[10,19,25,31] Appropriate medication for anxiety or depression may secondarily influence SIT in a positive or negative manner.

Anxiety or depression is frequently associated with SIT. The stress diathesis model for depression has been translated to understand the anxiety and depression associated with tinnitus (SIT).[8,22,23] Specifically, increasing stress results in the clinical manifestation of anxiety and, over time, depression. The chronic nature of SIT suggests long-term treatment. Psychiatric consultation is advised to take advantage of the experience of the professional involved for anxiety and depression. Drug selection is at the discretion of the psychiatrist or psychologist. Anxiolytic and antidepressive medications, when recommended, may result in tinnitus. Medications involving neurotransmitter systems other than that of the involved drug in question are then to be used in drug selection Significant in the literature are reports that when anxiolytic or antidepressant medication is reported to be associated with tinnitus production or to increase the intensity of tinnitus, withdrawal of the drug has resulted in elimination of the tinnitus. Treatment of the anxiety or depression is considered to be critical for the success of any and all attempts to treat the sensory component.

Instrumentation and Tinnitus Control

The authors' first-line recommendation is medication, followed by instrumentation.[10,26] Specifically, control of factors influencing the clinical course of the SIT must be achieved.

Instrumentation available consists of hearing aids; tinnitus masks or tinnitus instruments; and tinnitus retraining therapy (TRT), including low-level noise generators, tapes or compact disks of the masking or relaxation external electrical stimulation, and ultrahigh-frequency stimulation.[26,33,39,40]

There are many devices to choose from, and there is a rationale for choosing a specific device. Improved instrumentation provides an increased ability to fit patients who have tinnitus with near-normal hearing, mild high-frequency hearing losses, hyperacusis, and high-frequency tinnitus.

Masking, the substitution of one sound for another, was reintroduced by Vernon[68,69] for attempting tinnitus relief. The masking stimulus, an external noise, provides tinnitus relief by "covering up" the tinnitus. In the authors' experience, the masker continues to be an effective modality of tinnitus relief in patients who have SIT in whom the factors influencing the tinnitus (ie, aeration of the middle ear, SEH) have been identified and treated, in patients who have a predominantly cochlear type of tinnitus, and in patients who have a Feldmann type 1 masking curve. Additional increase in the masker effect can be obtained in selected patients who have SIT by its combination with a hearing aid (ie, tinnitus instrument).[70,71]

TRT is based on the concept that that acoustic, or acoustic-like, perceptions could be habituated to if they were not considered to be a harbinger of disease, danger, or mental stress. Habituation to many sensory experiences is an integral part of human behavior.[40] In the authors' experience, TRT is recommended when medication approaches are ineffective for tinnitus relief. TRT has been most effective for hyperacusis control.

Ultrahigh-frequency acoustic stimulation provides tinnitus relief in a selected group of patients who have SIT and have residual hearing in the ultrahigh-frequency range.[32,33,54]

Surgery and Transcortical Magnetic Stimulation

In general, the results of surgery for tinnitus relief are conflicting, and there is no specific surgical procedure for the control of any CTT at this time. Results have been more satisfactory for objective tinnitus than for SIT.

Significant tinnitus relief with intratympanic steroid therapy has been reported for a predominantly cochlear type of tinnitus.[72,73] Investigational human cortical electrical stimulation has reported tinnitus relief.[74,75] Transcortical magnetic stimulation in humans has been reported to provide transient tinnitus relief.[74,76] Another surgical approach, deep brain stimulation, involving direct electrical stimulation of structures deep in the brain, has been reported to provide tinnitus relief.[77]

Psychologic Issues of Tinnitus: Cognitive-Based Therapy

The significance of personality dynamics and coping mechanisms to patients' perception of sensations; their significance for tinnitus; and their clinical application for control of the factors of stress, anxiety, and depression have been recognized and reported since 1984.[78–80]

Clinically, the efficacy of treatment and control for SIT has been increased since 1979 by inclusion in the MATPP of the need to treat the sensory and affect behavioral components of the SIT complaint. The MATPP recognizes the significant role played by counseling in the overall result of tinnitus relief. Specifically, methods of treatment include support groups, crisis intervention, cognitive- or insight-oriented therapies, and psychiatric consultations. Such approaches are considered to be primarily supportive and adjunctive in nature.[80–89] Resistance on the part of the patient who has SIT to such care has delayed the efficacy of treatment directed primarily to the sensory component. A stable personality for the patient who has SIT is considered to be essential for any or all therapies targeting the sensory component of the SIT. When reporting the results of tinnitus relief with supportive therapies, it is necessary to specify the results for SIT. In the authors' experience, the efficacy of cognitive-based therapy (CBT) depends on the readiness of the patient to change his or her behavior and thinking process(es) for the tinnitus and for himself or herself.

CBT refers to the analysis and modification of patterns of behavior, points of view, and outlooks of patients developed as a result or in response to their environment. It is based on the cognitive theory of emotions that was first developed by Beck[81] in the late 1960s.

CBT strategies for tinnitus treatment are not a single form of treatment and include the following:

A. Behavioral modification
B. Environmental or situation modification
C. Modification of negative results on behavior secondary to environmental influences. Techniques include relaxation, hypnosis, and thought stopping, for example.

The following CBT techniques reported for tinnitus relief have been found to be of significance in the authors' approach to relief of SIT:

1. Anxiety and depression: Sweetow[82–85] introduced and adapted, specifically for SIT, the experiences reported by neuropsychiatrists or psychologists of CBT for

complaints of anxiety and depression. The methods are adjunctive to approaches for SIT management methods rather than a substitute for other recommended treatments. Emphasis is placed on management of the patient who has tinnitus rather than on tinnitus management or treatment. Such adjunctive approaches are geared toward an attitudinal adjustment regarding one's reaction to the tinnitus rather than toward alleviating the tinnitus itself.

2. Relaxation techniques[86]
3. Stress, fear, anxiety, and depression control[87,88]
4. Anxiety and pain control[89,90]
5. Incorporation of audiologic techniques for CBT, including sound enrichment[91]
6. Focus on education alone and a cognitive rationale[92,93]
7. Learning theory based on the habituation model[94]
8. Behavior and cognitive restructuring

The effects have been reported of an Internet-based CBT self-help treatment for tinnitus, similar to those described by Sweetow in 1995 in a traditional clinical setting "to identify and modify maladaptive behaviors and beliefs by means of behavioral change and cognitive restructuring."[79]

"Significant reductions in distress" were reported. A 3-month follow-up assessment reported the improvement to be maintained. In this study, 27.3% of patients were reported to have "reached the conservative criteria of clinically significant improvement;" this rate increased to 38.9% when "only those who completed treatment were considered." Significant is the lack of data in this report of the results specifically for SIT.

ALTERNATIVE METHODS

Alternative methods of therapy in the literature include acupuncture; psychotherapy; hypnotherapy; and the use of herbal, vitamin, Gingko biloba extract 761, and antioxidant drugs. In general, such methods have reported conflicting tinnitus relief results.[10,95–99]

FUTURE

Future treatment for SIT is awaiting translation of advances in auditory and neuroscience for tinnitus diagnosis and treatment. This should include pharmacology for tinnitus, identified as tinnitopharmacoproteogenomics, instrumentation, and surgery.[19,69–76,100]

The goal is to identify the neurobiology of tinnitus, to identify the kinetics of gene expression in the brain of patients who have SIT, to "personalize" drug therapy for a particular CTT, and to identify not only the kinetics of the genome but the specific function of the protein(s) involved in the patients who have SIT with different CTTs (ie, tinnitoproteogenomics).

The development of drugs focusing on tinnitus control is identified as tinnitopharmacogenomics, which is defined as pharmacology for tinnitus based on what is known of the genetic diversity and protein function(s) demonstrated by patients diagnosed with different CTTs.

Future identification of epilepsy genes is hypothesized to provide insight into the molecular basis of neuronal excitability and brain function, which should have application for a particular central type of tinnitus.

SUMMARY

Those who evaluate and attempt to help patients who have SIT are advised to learn about and keep abreast of developments in the field of palliative medicine. Palliation medicine is not an alternative to other ways of managing patients who have SIT but is an approach that includes compassion, understanding, and the use of a broad range of expertise in ways that help to alleviate the anguish of patients who are constantly or intermittently exposed to the annoyance of hearing sounds they do not want to hear.

Tinnitus relief (ie, palliation) is available for the patient who has SIT based on an accurate diagnosis of tinnitus and followed by combined therapy of instrumentation and medication. Although no cure is available at this time for tinnitus of any clinical type, protocols of diagnosis and treatment are available that, when completed, provide a basis for treatment selection.

As we professionals strive to reach the goal of a cure for all CTTs, the integration of principles of palliative care into existing protocols for tinnitus diagnosis and treatment, by providing a holistic, compassionate, symptomatic, and interdisciplinary approach for tinnitus relief, should result in respect, understanding, and compassion for the patient who has SIT and a significant degree of tinnitus relief. No longer should a patient who has tinnitus be told "to live with it."

ACKNOWLEDGMENTS

The authors gratefully acknowledge the support of the Martha Entenmann Tinnitus Research Center, Inc., Forest Hills, New York, for this educational effort.

REFERENCES

1. American Tinnitus Association. Information about tinnitus. Portland (OR): Tinnitus Today; 1979.
2. Shulman A. Medical evaluation. In: Shulman A, Tonndorf J, Feldmann H, et al, editors. Tinnitus diagnosis/treatment. Philadelphia: Lea and Febiger; 1991. p. 253–92.
3. Dorland's pocket medical dictionary. 22nd edition. W.B. Saunders Co: Philadelphia: London Toronto. p. 510.
4. Oxford textbook of palliative medicine. 3rd edition. Doyle D, Hanks G, Cherny, Calman K, editors.
5. Bulletin of the American College of Surgeons, vol. 90, No.8, 2005.
6. Kandel E. In search of memory: the emergence of a new science of mind. New York: W.W. Norton; 2006.
7. Baxter L, Phelps M, Mazziotta T, et al. Local glucose cerebral metabolic rates in obsessive-compulsive disorder. Arch Gen Psychiatry 1987;44:211–8.
8. Shulman A. A final common pathway for tinnitus—the medial temporal lobe system. Int Tinnitus J 1995;1(1):115–26.
9. Shulman A, Goldstein B. Tinnitus dyssynchrony/synchrony theory: a translational concept for tinnitus diagnosis and treatment. Int Tinnitus J 2006;12(2):101–14.
10. Shulman A, Tonndorf J, Feldmann H, et al. Tinnitus diagnosis treatment. Philadelphia: Lea B Febiger; 1991.
11. Shulman A. Subjective idiopathic tinnitus clinical types: a system of nomenclature and classification. In: Feldmann H, editor. Proceedings of the Third International Tinnitus Seminar. Karlsruhe: Harsch Verlag, 1987: 136–41.
12. Shulman A. Subclinical tinnitus: non-auditory tinnitus. Br J Laryngol Otol Suppl 1984;9:77–9.

13. Shulman A. Secondary endolymphatic hydrops. AAOHNS Transactions 1991; 104(NO.1):146–7 Mosby Co. 1/91.
14. Erlandsson SI, Hallberg LR-M. Prediction of quality of life in patients with tinnitus. Br J Audiol 2000;34(9):11–9.
15. Nondahl D, Cruickshanks KJ, Dalton DS, et al. The impact of tinnitus on quality of life in older adults. J Am Acad Audiol 2007;18(3):257–66.
16. Shulman A. Speculations and conclusions. In: Shulman A, Aran JM, Feldmann H, et al, editors. Tinnitus diagnosis/treatment. Philadelphia: Lea and Febiger; 1991.
17. Shulman A. Tinnitus diagnosis/treatment. Hear Aid J 1979;32–4.
18. Shulman A. Clinical types of tinnitus. In: Shulman A, Tonndorf J, Feldmann H, et al, editors. Tinnitus diagnosis/treatment. Philadelphia: Lea and Febiger; 1991. p. 323–41.
19. Shulman A, Goldstein B. Pharmacotherapy for severe disabling subjective idiopathic tinnitus. Int Tinnitus J 2006;12(2):161–71.
20. Feldmann H. Homolateral and contralateral masking of tinnitus by noise bands and pure tones. Audiology,10:138–144.
21. Somjen G. Sensory coding in the mammalian nervous system. New York: Appleton-Century-Crofts; 1972.
22. Shulman A. Stress model for tinnitus. Presentation International Tinnitus Group. Washington DC; 1992.
23. Shulman A. Stress model for tinnitus. Neurotol Newsletter 1998;3(3):53–7.
24. Shulman A, Goldstein B. Medical significance tinnitus. Int Tinnitus J 1997;3(1): 45–50.
25. Shulman A. Medical methods, drug therapy, and tinnitus control strategies. In: Shulman A, Tonndorf J, Feldmann H, editors. Tinnitus diagnosis/treatment. Philadelphia: Lea and Febiger; 1991. p. 453–89.
26. Shulman A. Instrumentation. In: Shulman A, Tonndorf J, Feldmann H, editors. Tinnitus diagnosis/treatment. Philadelphia: Lea and Febiger; 1991. p. 503–13.
27. Descartes R. The philosophical writings of Descartes, 3 vols. Translated by John Cottingham, Robert Stoothoff and Dugald Murdoch, volume 3 including Anthony Kenny. In Meditations 1,2,6. Cambridge: Cambridge University Press, 1988.
28. Shulman A. Medical audiologic tinnitus patient protocol. In: Shulman A, et al, editors. Tinnitus diagnosis/treatment. Philadelphia: Lea & Febiger; 1991. p. 319.
29. Daftary A, Shulman A, Strashun AM, et al. Benzodiazepine receptor distribution in severe disabling tinnitus. Int Tinnitus J 2004;10(1):17–23.
30. Shulman A, Goldstein B, Avitable MJ. Quantitative electroencephalography-power analysis. A electrophysiologic correlate of brain function in subjective idiopathic tinnitus patients. (N-61). A clinical paradigm shift in the understanding of tinnitus. Int Tinnitus J 2006;12(2):121–32.
31. Shulman A, Strashun AM, Goldstein BA. GABA A–benzodiazepine—chloride receptor-targeted therapy for tinnitus control: preliminary report. Int Tinnitus J 2002;8:30–6.
32. Lenhardt ML, Skellett R, Wang P, et al. Human ultrasonic speech perception. Science 1991;253:82–5.
33. Goldstein BA, Shulman A, Lenhardt ML, et al. Long-term inhibition of tinnitus by UltraQuiet therapy: preliminary report. Int Tinnitus J 2001;7(2):122–7.
34. Shulman A. Tinnitology, tinnitogenesis, nuclear medicine, and tinnitus patients. Int Tinnitus J 1998;4(2):102–8.
35. Eggermont JJ. Tinnitus: some thoughts about its origin. J Laryngol Otol 1984;(Suppl 9):31–7.

36. Eggermont JJ. On the pathophysiology of tinnitus: a review and a peripheral model. Hear Res 1990;48:11–124.
37. Moller A. Pathophysiology of tinnitus. Ann Otol Rhinol Laryngol 1984;93:39–44.
38. Tonndorf J. The analogy between tinnitus and pain. A suggestion for a physiological basis for chronic tinnitus. Hear res 1997;28:271–5.
39. Jastreboff PJ. Phantom auditory perception (tinnitus): mechanisms of generation and perception. Neurosci Res 1990;8:22–254.
40. Jastreboff PJ, Hazell JWP. A neurophysiological approach to tinnitus: clinical implications. Br J Audiol 1993;27:7–17.
41. Stylpkowski PH. Physiological mechanisms of salicylate ototoxicity. Hear Res 1990;46:113–45.
42. LePage EL. Frequency dependent self induced bias of the basilar membrane and its potential for controlling sensitivity and tuning in the mammalian cochlea. J Acoust Soc Am 1987;82:139–54.
43. Moller AR. Can injury to the auditory nerve cause tinnitus? In: Feldmann H, editor. Proceedings of the III International Tinnitus Seminar, 58–63 Karlsruhe, Harsch Verlag; 1987.
44. Hazel JWP. A cochlear model for tinnitus. In: Feldmann H, editor. Proceedings of the Third International Tinnitis Seminar. Meunster, 121–128, Karlsruhe, Harsch Verlag. 1987.
45. Shulman A. Efferent auditory pathways and tinnitus. In: Shulman A, Aran JM, Feldman H, et al, editors. Tinnitus diagnosis/treatment. Philadelphia: Lea & Febiger; 1991. p. 184–210.
46. Brown MC, Berglund AM, Kiang NY-S, et al. Central trajectories of Type II spiral ganglion neurons. J Comp Neurol 1988;278:581–90.
47. Claussen CF, Franz B. Contemporary and practical neurotology. Hanover: Pharmaceuticals, Solvay Pharmaceuticals, GmbH; 2006.
48. Claussen CF. Die Cranio-Corpo-graphie (CCG), eine einfache Photooptische Registrierungsmethode fur Vestibulospinale Reaktionen. Zeitschr Laryngol Rhinol 1970;49:6–639.
49. Shulman A, Strashun AM, et al. Descending auditory system/cerebellum/tinnitus. Int Tinnitus J 1999;5(2):92–106.
50. Shulman A, Strashun AM, Goldstein BA, et al. Neurospect cerebral blood flow studies in patients with a central type tinnitus. Preliminary study. In: Transactions of the Fourth International Tinnitus Seminar, Amsterdam Kugler Public. 1991:211–5.
51. Shulman A, Strashun AM, Afriyie M, et al. SPECT imaging of brain and tinnitus—neurotology neurologic implications. Int Tinnitus J 1995;1(1):13–29.
52. Shulman A, Strashun AM, Seibyl JP, et al. Benzodiazepine receptor deficiency and tinnitus. Int Tinnitus J 2000;6(2):98–111.
53. Shulman A, Strashun AM, Avitable MJ, et al. Ultrahigh frequency acoustic stimulation and tinnitus control—a PET study. Int Tinnitus J 2004;10(2).
54. Goldstein B, Shulman A. Tinnitus—hyperacusis and the loudness discomfort test: a preliminary report. Int Tinnitus J 1996;2(1):83–9.
55. Shulman A, Seitz M. Central tinnitus—diagnosis/treatment. Observations of simultaneous binaural auditory brainstem responses with monaural stimulation in the tinnitus patient. Laryngoscope 1981;912025–35.
56. Shulman A. Auditory brainstem response and tinnitus. In: Shulman A, Tonndorf J, Feldmann H, editors. Tinnitus diagnosis/treatment. Philadelphia: Lea B Febiger; 1991. p. 138–83.

57. Itard JMG. Traites des maladies de l'orielle et de l'audition. Paris: Mequignon-Maarvis; 1821.
58. Llinas R, Urbano FJ, et al. Rhythmic and dysrhythmic thalamocortical dynamics: GABA systems and the edge effect. Trends in Neurosciences. 2005;28(6):325–33.
59. Jastreboff P. Tinnitus as a phantom perception: theories and clinical implications. In: Vernon JA, Moller AR, editors. Mechanisms of tinnitus. Allyn and Bacon; 1995. p. 73–87.
60. Uttal WR. Emerging principles of sensory coding. In: Uttal WR, editor. Sensory coding—selected readings. Boston: Little,Brown & Co; 1972.
61. Shulman A. External electrical tinnitus suppression: a review. 1983–1985. Am J Otol 1987;8:479–84.
62. Shulman A. Electrodiagnostics, electrotherapeutics, and other approaches to the management of tinnitus. In: AAO-HNS instructional courses, vol. 11. St. Louis: C.V. Mosby; 1989. p. 137.
63. Steenerson RL, Cronin GW. Electrical stimulation in the treatment of tinnitus. In: Reich GE, Vernon JA, editors. Proceedings of the Fifth International Tinnitus Seminar 1995. Portland, OR: American Tinnitus Association; 1996:353–6.
64. Rubinstein JT, Tyler RS, Johnson A, et al. Electrical suppression tinnitus with high rate pulse trains. Otol Neurotol 2003;24(3):478–85.
65. Vernon JA, Schleuning AJ. Tinnitus: a new management. Laryngoscope 1978;85: 413–9.
66. Vernon J. The use of masking in relief of tinnitus. In: Silverstein H, Norell H, editors. Neurological surgery of the ear. Birmingham, AL: Aesculapius; 1979.
67. Shulman A, Goldstein B. Tinnitus masking—a longitudinal study of efficacy diagnosis: treatment 1977–1986. In: Feldmann H, editor. Proceedings of the Third International Tinnitus Seminar. Karlsruhe, Harsch Verlag, 1987:251–6.
68. Goldstein B, Shulman A. Tinnitus masking—a longitudinal study 1987–1994. In: Reich GE, Vernon JA, editors. Proceedings of the Fifth International Tinnitus Seminar 1995. Portland, OR: American Tinnitus Association; 1996. p. 315–21.
69. De Ridder D, De Mulder G, Walsh V, et al. Magnetic and electrical stimulation of the auditory cortex for intractable tinnitus. Case report. J Neurosurg 2004;100(3):560–4.
70. De Ridder D, De Mulder G, Verstraeten E, et al. Auditory cortex stimulation for tinnitus. Acta Neurochir Suppl 2007;97(Pt 2):451–62.
71. Dornhoffer JL, Mennemeier M. Transcranial magnetic stimulation and tinnitus: implications for theory and practice. J Neurol Neurosurg Psychiatr 2007;78:113.
72. Shiy YB, Martin WH. Deep grain stimulation—a new treatment of tinnitus? In: Proceedings of the Sixth International Tinnitus Seminar. CD Rom, Tinnitus & Hyperacusis Centre, London.
73. House PR. Personality of the tinnitus patient. In: Shulman A, Ballantine J, editors. Proceedings of the Second International Tinnitus Seminar. Laryngol. Otol. Suppl; 1984,9:233–5.
74. Aldo-Sandstrom K, Larsen HC, Andersson G. Internet-based cognitive-behavioral self-help treatment of tinnitus: clinical effectiveness and predictors of outcome. Am J Audiol 2004;13:185–92.
75. Shulman A. Psychological issues of tinnitus. In: Shulman A, Tonndorf J, Feldmann H, editors. Tinnitus diagnosis/treatment. Philadelphia: Lea and Febiger; 1991. p. 533–7.
76. Beck AT. Cognitive therapy and the emotional disorders. New York: International University Press; 1976.
77. Sweetow RW. The support education group approach to coping with tinnitus. In: Clark JG, Anick PY, editors. Tinnitus and its management. Springfield (IL): Charles C. Thomas; 1984.

78. Sweetow R. Cognitive aspects of tinnitus patient management. Ear Hear 1986; 7(6):390–6.
79. Sweetow R. Adjunctive approaches to tinnitus—patient management. Hear J 1989;42(11):38–44.
80. Sweetow RW. The evolution of cognitive-behavioral therapy as an approach to tinnitus management. Int Tinnitus J 1995;1:61–5.
81. Lindberg P, Scott B, Melin L, et al. Behavioral therapy in the clinical management of tinnitus. Br J Audiol 1988;22:265–72.
82. Wayner DS. A cognitive therapy weekend workshop for tinnitus: a followup report. In: Vernon JA, Reich GE, editors. Proceeding of the Fifth International Tinnitus Seminar. American Tinnitus Association; 1996. p. 607–10.
83. Wayner DS. A cognitive therapy and tinnitus: a workshop manual. Portland, (OR): American Tinnitus Association; 1991.
84. Barlow DH. Clinical handbook of psychological disorders. A step-by-step treatment manual. 3rd edition. New York: Guilford Press; 2001.
85. Philips HC, Rachman S. The psychological management of pain. New York: Springer; 1996.
86. Haerkotter C, Hiller W. (2002) Combining elements of tinnitus retraining therapy (TRT) and cognitive-behavioral therapy: does it work? In: Pattucci R, editor. Proceedings of the Seventh International Tinnitus Seminar. p. 7, Fremantle: University of Western Australia.
87. Henry JL, Wilson PH. Psychological management of tinnitus: comparison of a combined cognitive educational program, education alone, and a waiting list control. Int Tinnitus J 1996;2(1):11–2.
88. Alpini D, Caesarani A, Hahn A. Tinnitus school: an educational approach to tinnitus management based on a stress-reaction tinnitus model. Int Tinnitus J 2007;13(1):63–8.
89. Hallam RS, Rachman S, Hinchcliffe R. Psychological aspects of tinnitus. In: Rachman S, editor. Contributions to medical psychology, vol. 3. Oxford (UK): Pergamon Press; 1984. p. 31–53.
90. Seidman MD, Van De Water TR. Pharmacologic manipulation of the labyrinth with novel and traditional agents delivered to the inner ear. Ear Nose Throat J 2003;82:279–80, 282–3, 287–8.
91. Shulman A. Biofeedback. In: Shulman A, Tonndorf J, Feldmann H, editors. Tinnitus diagnosis/treatment. Philadelphia: Lea & Febiger; 1991. p. 538–9.
92. Shulman A. Hypnotherapy. In: Shulman A, Tonndorf J, Feldmann H, editors. Tinnitus diagnosis/treatment. Philadelphia: Lea & Febiger; 1991. p. 540–1.
93. Kitahara M. Combined treatment for tinnitus. In: Kitahara M, editor. Tinnitus, pathophysiology and management. Tokyo: Igaku-Shoin; 1988. p. 107–17.
94. Shulman A. Neuroprotective drug therapy: a medical and pharmacological treatment for tinnitus control. Int Tinnitus J 1997;3(2):77–94.
95. Shulman A. Tinnitus neural substrates: an addendum. Int Tinn J 2005;11(1):1–3.
96. Pillsbury HL. Hyertension, hyperlipidemia, chronic noise exposure. Is there synergism in cochlear pathology? Laryngoscope 1986;96:1112–38.
97. Brookler KH. Etidronate for neurotologic symptoms of otosclerosis. Ear Nose Throat J 2002;76(6):371–6.
98. Sakata E, Itoh A, Ohtsu K, et al. Treatment of cochlear tinnitus. Effect of transtympanic infusion with dexamethasone fluid. Audiology (jpn) 1983;26:148–51.
99. Shulman A, Goldstein B. Intratympanic drug therapy with steroids for tinnitus control: a preliminary report. Int Tinnitus J 2000;6(1):10–20.
100. Seidman MD, DeRidder D, Elisovich K, et al. Direct Electrical Stimulation of Heschel's Gyrus for Tinnitus Treatment. Laryngoscope 2008;118:491–500.

Palliative Care for the Patient with Refractory Chronic Rhinosinusitis

Elizabeth J. Mahoney, MD[a],*, Ralph Metson, MD[b]

KEYWORDS

- Rhinosinusitis • Refractory • Palliative

Chronic rhinosinusitis (CRS) is a chronic condition affecting 14% to 16% of the United States population.[1] Patients with CRS have been shown to have a significant decrement in their quality of life, including domains of physical and social functioning.[2] Although well-established therapeutic options are available for the treatment of CRS, there remains a subset of patients with this disorder who fail to demonstrate symptomatic improvement following conventional therapy. For the patients who have failed to achieve relief of symptoms of CRS after both medical and surgical treatment, often there is a need for some kind of continuing care and usually the otolaryngologist is the member of the health care team to whom the responsibility falls for providing this continuing care, especially for those patients who have already had sinus surgery. In a sense, perhaps unwittingly, the otolaryngologist is providing palliative care when continuing to care for the patient who is having symptoms of CRS after medical and surgical management has been tried. By definition, palliative care attempts to help a patient live reasonably well with a medical condition that cannot be completely eradicated. To provide such care to the CRS patient, the otolaryngologist needs to be creative in devising treatment regimens customized to the unique needs of each patient.

THE SINUSITIS SPECTRUM

CRS has been defined by the Sinus and Allergy Health Partnership as a group of disorders characterized by inflammation of the nasal and paranasal sinus mucosa of at least 12 consecutive weeks' duration.[3] This chronic disorder can be viewed as a spectrum of pathology, ranging from localized processes to systemic disorders. Understanding this "sinusitis spectrum" may be helpful in identifying those patients at

[a] Department of Otolaryngology—Head and Neck Surgery, Boston University School of Medicine, F.G.H. Building, 820 Harrison Avenue, One Boston Medical Center Place, Boston, MA 02118, USA
[b] Department of Otology and Laryngology, Harvard Medical School, Zero Emerson Place, Boston, MA 02114, USA
* Corresponding author.
E-mail address: Elizabeth.mahoney@bmc.org (E.J. Mahoney).

Otolaryngol Clin N Am 42 (2009) 39–47
doi:10.1016/j.otc.2008.09.009
0030-6665/08/$ – see front matter © 2009 Elsevier Inc. All rights reserved.

oto.theclinics.com

increased risk for failing conventional therapies, and in tailoring the treatment approach to fit a patient's individual needs.

At one end of the sinusitis spectrum is the patient with "local" disease. These patients tend to have clear anatomic factors predisposing toward sinus infection. Anatomic obstructions, such as conchae bullosae and septal deviations, are examples of local factors that may obstruct normal mucociliary flow. Additionally, patients with an isolated polyp or neoplasm may be classified as having local disease. Such local factors can usually be readily identified on nasal endoscopy or sinus imaging, and can be routinely addressed with conventional endoscopic surgical approaches.

At the other end of the sinusitis spectrum are those patients with "systemic" disease. These patients have an underlying systemic disorder leading to diffuse inflammation of the sinonasal mucosa, often with polyp formation, which places them at heightened risk for recurrent sinus infections. Individuals who may be classified in this category include those with triad asthma, granulomatous disease, cystic fibrosis, immunodeficiency, and primary ciliary dyskinesia. These systemic patients are at highest risk for failing conventional medical and surgical therapies used to treat CRS.

Within this sinusitis spectrum, there are a large number of patients who fall somewhere in the middle, between locals and systemics. This group of patients is referred to as "intermediates." They may have a combination of localized and systemic disease. Many of these patients, however, when treated with standard medical and surgical therapies, fare quite well (**Fig. 1**).

PATHOPHYSIOLOGY

Traditionally, CRS was understood to be the end stage of a disease process characterized by multiple acute bacterial infections. This theory, however, has been supplanted by the recognition that CRS is characterized by an aberrant inflammatory response in the sinonasal mucosa.[3] Although initiating events may vary, it is well understood that inflammation causing mucosal obstruction at sinus ostia triggers a cascade of events including impaired mucociliary clearance with stasis and bacterial overgrowth. In the absence of systemic disease, such as cystic fibrosis or an immune deficiency, a number of different paradigms have been postulated to explain the heightened sinonasal inflammatory response seen in CRS.

Although controversy exists as to whether bacteria play a direct or indirect role in the pathophysiology of CRS, antibiotic therapy remains a mainstay of treatment. Theories to explain how the presence of bacteria within the paranasal sinuses may trigger a non-infectious inflammatory process include the superantigen and biofilm theories.

It has long been recognized that certain bacteria secrete proteins called exotoxins, which are damaging to the host organism. A superantigen is a highly potent exotoxin that has been associated with dramatic disease processes, such as the toxic shock syndrome triggered by *Staphylococcus aureus'* production of superantigen. Recent

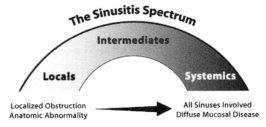

Fig. 1. The sinusitis spectrum.

interest has focused on the potential role of superantigens in triggering sinonasal inflammation. A recent study by Bernstein and colleagues[4] demonstrated toxin-producing S aureus in the nasal mucus adjacent to polyps in 55% of patients with chronic hyperplastic sinusitis and nasal polyposis. The corresponding variable β T-cell receptor site was also noted to be up-regulated. Although an understanding of the superantigen link to CRS continues to evolve, it seems that microbial superantigens bind to T-cell receptors and major histocompatibility complex II molecules in a fashion that bypasses the typical route of antigen presentation, resulting in an enhanced activation of the host T-cell population.[5] This cascade results in massive cytokine release and eosinophilic activation with consequent mucosal insult and inflammation.

The biofilm theory has also been postulated to explain the pathologic role of bacteria in the CRS process. Biofilms are created when bacteria bind to a surface and generate a community of microorganisms in a matrix attached to a surface. Bacteria in a biofilm state have a reduced metabolic state and do not provoke the exuberant systemic response elicited by free-floating bacteria. They demonstrate decreased susceptibility to systemic and local antibiotic therapy. In addition, they intermittently release free-floating bacteria that can serve as a continuous nidus of infection. Although biofilms have been identified on the surface of sinus mucosa of patients with CRS, the significance of these biofilms remains a subject of continued investigation.[6,7]

Atopic disease is also recognized as playing a key role in the pathophysiology of CRS. Although the epidemiologic association between CRS and allergy is well established, a causal relationship remains more elusive. In one study that examined the presence of allergy among patients undergoing functional endoscopic sinus surgery, 80% of patients were noted to have elevated specific IgE levels.[8] These epidemiologic observations, however, fail to provide an explanation of the causal relationship between allergy and CRS. One mechanism that may help to explain such a causal relationship is the induction of mucosal edema and sinus ostia obstruction through the release of allergic mediators and cytokines. Additionally, it has been shown that in patients undergoing sinus surgery, surgical outcomes are enhanced by treatment of underlying inhalant allergy.[9]

Allergic fungal sinusitis has emerged as a clinically distinct subset of CRS, and merits special consideration in this discussion. Diagnostic criteria for allergic fungal sinusitis include eosinophilic mucin-containing noninvasive fungal hyphae and Charcot-Leyden crystals on microscopic examination. Patients with this disorder typically present with nasal polyposis, characteristic radiographic findings, immunocompetence, and allergy.[10] Although theories to explain the phenomenon of allergic fungal sinusitis abound, the core principle is based on the premise that it is the inflammatory response to fungus, rather than the mere presence of fungus. In 1999, the concept of a nonallergic fungal inflammatory process was described by Ponikau and coworkers[11] who identified hyphae in over 90% of patients with CRS. Eosinophils were also noted to be migrating into the mucus in characteristic clusters. In this study population, allergy to fungus failed to correlate with CRS. The suggested terminology was changed from allergic fungal rhinosinusitis to eosinophilic fungal rhinosinusitis. Questions and controversy continue to surround the significance of fungi in CRS.

WHY PATIENTS FAIL TO FIND THE RELIEF THEY ARE SEEKING

Understanding pathophysiologic events that may lead to CRS helps the otolaryngologist to understand why certain patients may fail conventional therapy. Maximal medical therapy typically involves courses of antimicrobials, nasal steroid sprays, and possibly systemic steroids. Antihistamines, decongestants, and mucous thinning agents may also be used in selected patients. Sinus surgery is typically offered to patients who fail to respond to these measures and excellent success rates ranging from 80% to 90% have been reported.[12,13] Despite the success noted with functional endoscopic sinus surgery, there exists a subset of patients who do not improve after one or more endoscopic sinus procedures, even when postoperative nasal endoscopy and CT scan show patent sinus ostia. For the purpose of this discussion, conventional therapy is defined as the use of the previously mentioned medical therapies and patient-appropriate surgical interventions.

Although it may seem obvious, possible anatomic explanations for such failure should be investigated. Areas of synechiae and cicatricial scarring should be sought on CT and nasal endoscopy. Patients with recurrent nasal polyposis are at high risk for failed therapy as the polyps continue to grow and become a source of anatomic obstruction. More radical surgery, such as a frontal sinus drillout or obliteration, may be necessary for the otolaryngologist to consider in select patients.

In addition to an anatomic evaluation, such patients should have a thorough medical evaluation, which may require a multidisciplinary approach. Patients should be evaluated for systemic disorders that may account for failed therapy, such as immunodeficiency, allergy, Samters triad, granulomatous disease, vasculitides, ciliary dyskinesia, and cystic fibrosis. It is this patient population with systemic disease that often becomes the most refractory to standard surgical and medical therapy. At this point, a change in focus toward palliative care may be helpful.

TREATMENT OPTIONS

Palliative care by no means implies avoidance of aggressive medical or surgical therapy. Rather, palliative care implies the provision of care that allows the patient to live with his or her disease in a state aimed at preservation of quality of life. Multidisciplinary therapies whose goal is symptomatic improvement, and novel and experimental therapeutic regimens, are reasonable to consider when a patient has exhausted conventional treatment options.

Immunomodulatory Therapy

An assessment for immunodeficiency should be performed in patients with CRS refractory to conventional medical treatment. Interestingly, among a group of 78 patients with refractory sinusitis at a tertiary care facility, 17.9% were noted to have low IgG and 16.7% were noted to have low IgA. Common variable immunodeficiency was diagnosed in 9.9% and selective IgA deficiency was found in 6.2%.[14] Sethi and colleagues[15] recommend that the minimum immunologic evaluation in patients with CRS refractory to conventional medical therapy should include measurements of quantitative immunoglobulin and IgG subclass levels, complete blood count with differential, and responses to immunization with protein and polysaccharide antigens. Such assessment for subtle immunodeficiency is important, because intravenous immune globulin infusions are often beneficial in patients with deficiencies of IgG. Nevertheless, extending the standard application of intravenous immune globulin therapy for the treatment of recalcitrant sinusitis remains controversial. One open-trial study of intravenous immune globulin in six patients suggested the efficacy of monthly intravenous immune globulin as an adjunctive treatment in patients with chronic sinusitis who failed conventional medical management. The protocol involved a 12-month trial of monthly intravenous immune globulin infusions (400 mg/kg). Five of six patients had decreased antibiotic use and the total number of sinusitis episodes also decreased.

These findings correlated with radiographic improvement in sinus disease.[16] More recently, subcutaneous IgG replacement therapy has been introduced, allowing for administration of similar cumulative doses at home.[17] Preliminary data suggest similar efficacy in protection against infection; however, this modality of treatment has yet to be evaluated in patients with CRS.

Leukotriene inhibitors including montelukast, zafirlukast, and zileuton have been shown to reduce both peripheral blood eosinophil counts and tissue eosinophilia in asthmatics. The same effect is believed to occur in CRS patients.[18] Leukotriene inhibitors have been shown to be effective in the treatment of CRS in open-label studies, particularly in patients with nasal polyposis and asthma. In a small prospective study, a statistically significant benefit for montelukast treatment in patients with nasal polyposis was observed both by symptom scores and polyp eosinophil counts.[19]

Aspirin desensitization has also been shown to down-regulate the cysL1-receptor expression and may have a role in the treatment of patients with refractory nasal polyposis and aspirin sensitivity. More specifically, aspirin desensitization may be indicated for patients who have aspirin-exacerbated respiratory disease and rhinosinusitis refractory to inhaled corticosteroids and leukotriene inhibitors. After initial desensitization, the maintenance of aspirin desensitization requires daily aspirin typically given at 650 mg twice-a-day doses. The daily dosing is very important, because subsequent desensitization is recommended if aspirin is missed for more than 48 hours.[20] The efficacy of aspirin desensitization therapy is supported by objective measures, which show a reduction in the number of sinus operations per year and sinus infections per year in patients who receive this treatment.[21]

Systemic Antibiotic Therapy

Consultation with an infectious disease specialist may be of benefit for consideration of less conventional antibiotic dosing regimens in refractory CRS patients. In one study, Anand and colleagues[22] demonstrated improved infection control in a group of patients with severe sinusitis who received up to 6 weeks of intravenous antibiotics based on pretreatment and posttreatment endoscopic culture results. Because of the difficulty in maintaining peripheral intravenous access for long intervals, oral antibiotics are more commonly used when treatment for several months is anticipated. To reduce the incidence of side effects and microbial resistance, the use of a lower than usual antibiotic dosage for long-term therapy has been advocated. Amoxicillin-clavulanate prescribed as a single daily dose of 500 mg, rather than the usual twice-a-day dosing, is practiced by some physicians. Although there is limited evidence to support the use of these regimens for chronic sinusitis, several studies have demonstrated the efficacy of low-dose, long-term antimicrobials for the treatment of recurrent episodes of otitis media in children.[23,24]

Long-term low-dose macrolide therapy may also be considered for its anti-inflammatory effect. Distinct from their antimicrobial properties, macrolides have been shown to have an anti-inflammatory effect and recent studies have shown that they may be effective in treating chronic airway inflammation, including the inflammation seen in CRS. Although the mechanism of macrolides' anti-inflammatory effects is not entirely understood, they seem to down-regulate proinflammatory cytokines and inhibit migration of inflammatory cells.[25] A recent study by Wallwork and colleagues[26] supports the practice of prescribing daily macrolides in patients with recalcitrant CRS. In a double-blind, randomized, placebo-controlled trial, patients who received 150 mg roxithromycin daily were found to have a statistically significant improvement in Sinonasal Outcome Test-20 scores and nasal endoscopy.

Topical Antibiotic Therapy

Topical antibiotics delivered to the nasal and sinus cavities have been widely used for the palliative treatment of patients with refractory sinusitis. These medications are typically delivered in liquid form as saline irrigations or in aerosolized droplets by a hand-held nebulizer. The potential advantage of topical therapy is that the antibiotic can be delivered in relatively high concentrations locally to the affected tissues, reducing the potential for systemic side effects. One noncontrolled study demonstrated the efficacy of culture-directed nebulized antibiotics in the treatment of acute sinusitis exacerbations in patients with CRS who had previously undergone functional endoscopic sinus surgery.[27] In a more recent review of clinical and basic science literature on the treatment of CRS with antimicrobial washes, Elliott and Stringer[28] recommend that topical antimicrobials be used in a culture-directed fashion. Normal saline is the typical delivery vehicle. Topical antibiotics are most commonly used in patients with a history of sinus surgery, because it is believed that the ability of topical antibiotics to reach the interior of sinus cavities may be contingent on the presence of surgically opened sinus ostia.

A number of antibiotic agents, including levofloxacin, tobramycin, and ceftazidime, are commercially available in preparations suitable for nebulized delivery. Although no topical antibiotics are approved by the Food and Drug Administration (FDA) for delivery into the nasal cavity, many such preparations have been compounded by local pharmacies for years. Antibiotic powder dissolved in saline for intravenous administration can be placed in a spray bottle for nasal applications. This liquid medication can also be squirted directly into the nose and sinuses by a soft plastic bulb syringe or squeeze bottle.

Neurologic Evaluation

For the patient with persistent headache and facial pain following CRS therapy, involvement of a neurologist or pain specialist as part of the treatment team may prove helpful. It is important for the consultant to rule out comorbid diagnoses, such as migraine, atypical facial pain syndrome, fibromyalgia, and neuralgia. Failure to recognize these diagnoses may confuse the otolaryngologist's interpretation of the patient's symptoms and lead to suboptimal patient care. Depending on the neurologic diagnosis, various treatment options are available to mitigate the patient's discomfort. In addition to a variety of available antimigraine medications, the use of antiepileptic medications, including gabapentin and topiramate, and antidepressant medications, such as amitriptyline, has demonstrated efficacy for treatment of patients with neuropathic pain. Although not FDA-approved for such use, the use of botulinum toxin (Botox) injected subcutaneously into pain trigger points in the head and neck has been shown to be effective in the treatment of select patients with atypical facial pain.[29]

Saline Irrigations

Maintenance of proper nasal hygiene with nasal saline irrigations is a mainstay of treatment in the patient with CRS and can be particularly beneficial when palliative therapy is needed. Cleansing the sinonasal membranes with salt water solution has been shown to facilitate mucociliary clearance and improve quality of life in such patients.[30] A recent Cochrane Review concluded that there is adequate evidence to support the use of saline irrigations as both a sole modality of treatment and adjunctive treatment for CRS.[31]

A variety of products and brands are commercially marketed for such use, including NeilMed Sinus Rinse, ENTSOL spray, and Saltaire. Most devices use a squeeze bottle, which is filled with saline solution. By gently squeezing the bottle, the solution is directed out a hole in the top of the bottle and into the patient's nostril. The solution then runs back out of the nostril as it carries with it mucus and debris that may be obstructing the nasal passages and sinuses. Most preparations contain isotonic saline solution, although some patients find hypertonic solutions to be more effective, particularly when the mucus is very thick. It is recommended that most patients irrigate twice a day, although more frequent usage is not harmful.

A saline solution can be prepared at home; however, many patients find the commercially available preparations to be more convenient, improving compliance with the prescribed regimen. The NetiPot is another means of nasal washing, which involves instillation of warm saline solution by a spouted pot. The spout of the pot is inserted into one nostril; the position of the head and pot are adjusted to allow the water to flow out of the other nostril. This technique is usually best suited for patients with thinner clear mucus and may not be as helpful in patients with thick tenacious mucus as is often seen in CRS.

Antifungal Therapy

Experimental use of intranasal antifungal agents has been reported as successful in the treatment of patients with CRS and should be given consideration. The premise of topical therapy is based on the theory that reduction of fungal antigenic load reduces eosinophilic activation and the subsequent release of inflammatory factors, which can lead to sinusitis. In a double-blind, placebo-controlled trial of daily intranasal instillation of amphotericin B, Ponikau and colleagues[32] showed an objective improvement in radiographic and endoscopic findings of CRS. These findings were questioned by Ebbens and colleagues[33] when a subsequent multicenter study of similar design failed to show significant differences between amphotericin and placebo groups in either subjective or objective outcome measures. Clearly, controversy continues to surround the issue of antifungal treatment for CRS.

FUTURE DIRECTIONS

In the future, treatment of patients with refractory CRS likely will include the use of newer immunomodulatory medications. Omalizumab, a monoclonal anti-IgE agent, has been noted to be effective in treating allergic asthma and allergic rhinitis.[34] Because of concerns about anaphylaxis, omalizumab currently has limited indications and is restricted to use in persons greater than 12 years of age with moderate to severe asthma who have a positive skin test or in vitro reactivity to a perennial aeroallergen and who have failed therapy with inhaled corticosteroids. The use of anti-interleukin agents, such as anti–interluekin-5, has also shown mixed results to date.[35,36]

Recent studies have begun to reveal a genetic basis for CRS through the use of DNA microarrays.[37,38] Genome-wide scanning of patients with sinusitis has identified the overexpression and underexpression of specific enzymes involved in the mucosal inflammation associated with CRS. The targeting of these aberrant genes and their protein products holds great promise for the future treatment of patients with sinusitis who remain symptomatic despite the best efforts of their treating physicians.

REFERENCES

1. Rosenfeld RM. Clinical practice guideline on adult sinusitis. Otolaryngol Head Neck Surg 2007;137(3):365–77.
2. Gliklich RE, Metson R. The health impact of chronic sinusitis in patients seeking otolaryngologic care. Otolaryngol Head Neck Surg 1995;113(1):104–9.

3. Benninger MS, Ferguson BJ, Hadley JA, et al. Adult chronic rhinosinusitis: definitions, diagnosis, epidemiology and pathophysiology. Otolaryngol Head Neck Surg 2003;129(3 Suppl):S1–32.

4. Bernstein JM, Ballow M, Schlievert PM, et al. A superantigen hypothesis for the pathogenesis of chronic hyperplastic sinusitis with massive nasal polyposis. Am J Rhinol 2003;17(6):321–6.

5. Seiberling KA, Grammer L, Kern RC. Chronic rhinosinusitis and superantigens. Otolaryngol Clin North Am 2005;38:1215–36.

6. Ferguson BJ, Stolz DB. Demonstration of biofilm in human bacterial chronic rhinosinusitis. Am J Rhinol 2005;19(5):452–7.

7. Sanderson AR, Leid JG, Hunsaker D. Bacterial biofilms on the sinus mucosa of human subjects with chronic rhinosinusitis. Laryngoscope 2006;116(7):1121–6.

8. Emaneul IA, Shah SB. Chronic rhinosinusitis: allergy and sinus computed tomography relationships. Otolaryngol Head Neck Surg 2000;123(6):687–91.

9. Nishioka GJ, Cook PR, Davis WE, et al. Immunotherapy in patients undergoing functional endoscopic sinus surgery. Otolaryngol Head Neck Surg 1994;110(4):406–12.

10. Bent JP, Kuhn FA. Diagnosis of allergic fungal sinusitis. Otolaryngol Head Neck Surg 1994;111(5):580–8.

11. Ponikau Ju, Sherris DA, Kern EB, et al. The diagnosis and incidence of allergic fungal sinusitis. Mayo Clin Proc 1999;74(9):877–84.

12. Senior BA, Kennedy DW, Tanabodee J, et al. Long-term results of functional endoscopic sinus surgery. Laryngoscope 1998;108(2):151–7.

13. King JM, Caldarelli DD, Pigato JB. A review of revision functional endoscopic sinus surgery. Laryngoscope Apr;104(4):404–8.

14. Chee L, Graham SM, Carother DG, et al. Immune dysfunction in refractory sinusitis in a tertiary care setting. Laryngoscope 2001;111(2):233–5.

15. Sethi DS, Winkelstein JA, Lederman H, et al. Immunologic defects in patients with chronic recurrent sinusitis: diagnosis and management. Otolaryngol Head Neck Surg 1995;112(2):242–7.

16. Ramesh S, Brodsky L, Afshani E, et al. Open trial of intravenous immune serum globulin for chronic sinusitis in children. Ann Allergy Asthma Immunol 1997; 79(2):119–24.

17. Gardulf A, Nicolay U, Asensio O, et al. Rapid subcutaneous IgG replacement therapy is effective and safe in children and adults with primary immunodeficiencies: a prospective, multi-national study. J Clin Immunol 2006;26(2):177–85.

18. Pizzichini E, Leff JA, Reiss TF, et al. Montelukast reduces airway eosinophilic inflammation in asthma: a randomized, controlled trial. Eur Respir J 1999;14:12–8.

19. Kieff DA, Busaba NY. Efficacy of montelukast in the treatment of nasal polyposis. Ann Otol Rhinol Laryngol 2005;114(12):941–5.

20. Macy E, Bernstein JA, Castells MC, et al. Aspirin challenge and desensitization for aspirin-exacerbated respiratory disease: a practice paper. Ann Allergy Asthma Immunol 2007;98(2):172–4.

21. Berges-Gimeno MP, Simon RA, Stevenson DD. Long-term treatment with aspirin desensitization in asthmatic patients with aspirin exacerbated respiratory disease. J Allergy Clin Immunol 2003;111(1):180–6.

22. Anand V, Levine H, Friedman M, et al. Intravenous antibiotics for refractory rhinosinusitis in nonsurgical patients: preliminary findings of a prospective study. Am J Rhinol 2003;17(6):363–8.

23. Marchisio P, Principi N, Sala E, et al. Comparative study of once-weekly azithromycin and once-daily amoxicillin treatments in prevention of recurrent otitis media in children. Antimicrobial Agents Chemother 1996;40(12):2732–6.
24. Paradise JL. Antimicrobial prophylaxis for recurrent acute otitis media. Ann Otol Rhinol Laryngol 1992;155:33–6.
25. Tamaoki J. The effects of macrolides on inflammatory cells. Chest 2004; 125(2 Suppl):41S–50S.
26. Wallwork B, Coman W, Mackay-Sim A, et al. A double-blind, randomized, placebo-controlled trial of macrolide in the treatment of chronic rhinosinusitis. Laryngoscope 2006;116(2):189–93.
27. Vaughan WC, Carvalho G. Use of nebulized antibiotics for acute infections in chronic sinusitis. Otolaryngol Head Neck Surg 2002;127(6):558–68.
28. Elliott KA, Stringer SP. Evidence-based recommendations for antimicrobial nasal washes in chronic rhinosinusitis. Am J Rhinol 2006;20(1):1–6.
29. Borodic GE, Acquadro M. The use of botulinum toxin for the treatment of chronic facial pain. J Pain 2002;3(1):21–7.
30. Tomooka LT, Murphy C, Davidson TM. Clinical study and literature review of nasal irrigation. Laryngoscope 2000;110(7):1189–93.
31. Burton MJ, Eisenberg LD, Rosenfeld RM. Extracts from The Cochrane Library: nasal saline irrigations for the symptoms of chronic rhinosinusitis. Otolaryngol Head Neck Surg 2007;137(4):532–4.
32. Ponikau JU, Sherris DA, Weaver A, et al. Treatment of chronic rhinosinusitis with intranasal amphotericin B: a randomized, placebo-controlled, double-blind pilot trial. J Allergy Clin Immunol 2005;115(1):125–31.
33. Ebbens FA, Scadding GK, Badia L, et al. Amphotericin B nasal lavages: not a solution for patients with chronic rhinosinusitis. J Allergy Clin Immunol 2006; 118(5):1149–56.
34. Vignola AM, Humbert M, Bousquet J, et al. Efficacy and tolerability of anti-immunoglobulin E therapy with omalizumab in patients with concomitant allergic asthma and persistent allergic rhinitis: SOLAR. Allergy 2004;59(7):709–17.
35. Leckie MJ, ten Brinke A, Khan J, et al. Effects of an interleukin-5 blocking monoclonal antibody on eosinophils, airway hyper-responsiveness, and the late asthmatic process. Lancet 2000;356(9248):2144–8.
36. Flood-Page PT, Menzies-Gow AN, Kay AB, et al. Eosinophil's role remains uncertain as anti-interleukin-5 only partially depletes numbers in the asthmatic airway. Am J Respir Crit Care Med 2003;167(2):199–204.
37. Liu Z, Kim J, Sypek JP, et al. Gene expression profiles in human nasal polyp tissues studied by means of DNA microarray. J Allergy Clin Immunol 2004;114(4): 783–90.
38. Fritz SB, Terrell JE, Conner ER, et al. Nasal mucosal gene expression in patients with allergic rhinitis with and without nasal polyps. J Allergy Clin Immunol 2003; 112(6):1057–63.

Rehabilitation After Cranial Base Surgery

Scharukh Jalisi, MD[a,b],*, James L. Netterville, MD[c]

KEYWORDS

• Voice • Dysphagia • Palliative • Cranial nerves • Rehabilitation

Not long ago, tumors of the cranial base were considered to be nonresectable, so a patient receiving the diagnosis of a skull base tumor was destined to die. However, with recent advancements in skull base surgery and with the advent of new and innovative modalities that can be used to remove or diminish the size of cranial base tumors, more than ever before can be done to preserve life for patients who have tumors in anatomic locations once considered unreachable without causing massive functional impairment. Nonetheless, modern-day resection of cranial base lesions still can be associated with significant perioperative complications and morbidity. The resulting outcome has a direct and serious impact on the quality of life of the patient. Advances in imaging techniques have enabled the detection of cranial base lesions at an early stage. Furthermore, new microsurgical and rehabilitative techniques not only allow resection of most cranial base tumors with preservation of cranial nerves and, hence, vital functions of the head and neck, but also allow for rehabilitative techniques that can help patients return to function faster. In this article on palliation, the authors focus on the rehabilitative techniques used in patients who have undergone extensive cranial base resection. These techniques can also be used to improve the life of patients who have not undergone surgery but suffer from poor quality of life because of the natural growth of the tumor.

EVALUATION

All patients undergoing cranial base resection undergo a thorough history and physical examination, including fiberoptic nasolaryngoscopy. Examination should focus on vocal fold motion, airway status, any pooling of secretions, and dysphagia. Appropriate imaging is obtained. It is advantageous to obtain a preoperative audiogram and

[a] Department of Otolaryngology—Head and Neck Surgery, Boston University Medical Center, 820 Harrison Avenue, FGH4, Boston, MA 02118, USA
[b] Department of Neurological surgery, Boston University Medical Center, 720 Harrison Avenue, Boston, MA 02118, USA
[c] Department of Otolaryngology—Head and Neck Surgery, Vanderbilt University, Medical Center East, 1215 21st Avenue, Nashville, TN 37232, USA
* Corresponding author. Department of Otolaryngology Head and Neck Surgery, Boston University Medical Center, Boston, MA.
E-mail address: sjalisi@bu.edu (S. Jalisi).

Otolaryngol Clin N Am 42 (2009) 49–56
doi:10.1016/j.otc.2008.09.016
0030-6665/08/$ – see front matter © 2009 Elsevier Inc. All rights reserved.

oto.theclinics.com

swallowing studies (modified barium swallow and functional endoscopic evaluation of swallowing and sensation). The latter can give important information about the pharyngeal and laryngeal sensation that is important in swallowing. The patient is evaluated using a multidisciplinary approach, including the head and neck surgeon, neurosurgeon, speech and language pathologist, audiologist, case management, and rehabilitation medicine.

CRANIAL NERVE DEFICITS
Olfactory Nerve (I)

The olfactory nerve carries special sensory afferents. The receptor neurons of the olfactory nerve are located in the upper part of the nasal cavity. These neurons continue to grow throughout life and get stimulated by gas molecules. The signal is transduced in the olfactory bulbs that lie in the cribriform plate. Anterior cranial base lesions such as olfactory neuroblastomas require resection of the cribriform plate and hence, the olfactory bulbs. Such patients need to be counseled about permanent postoperative anosmia. They are educated about using cooking gas at home because gas can leak and cause carbon dioxide/monoxide poisoning and can even be an explosion hazard. Therefore, these individuals need to have carbon dioxide and carbon monoxide detectors installed at home.

Optic Nerve (II)

The optic nerve has special sensory afferents. The optic nerve is resected during orbital exenteration or extensive tumor resection around the optic chiasm. In either situation, the nerve cannot be regenerated or grafted. The defect from the orbital exenteration, though, can be filled with prosthetics or obliterated with a vascularized local flap such as the temporoparietal fascial flap. Extensive defects that result in dural exposure are closed with vascularized free tissue transplantation.

Cavernous Sinus Nerves

The cavernous sinus contents include the oculomotor (III), the abducens (VI), and the first and second divisions of the trigeminal nerve (V1 and V2). Tumors involving this region can result in resection of these nerves.

The oculomotor nerve provides motor innervation to four extraocular muscles of the orbit: superior rectus, medial rectus, inferior oblique, and superior oblique. It also provides motor supply to the levator palpebrae superioris muscle and parasympathetic innervation to the ciliary muscles that constrict the pupil. Injury to this nerve results in inability to move the eye in all directions except laterally (abducens nerve) and inferomedially (trochlear nerve), upper eyelid ptosis, and the papillary dilation due to unopposed sympathetic action. The key rehabilitation in this case is of eyelid ptosis, which can be accomplished by levator tightening procedures to allow for the eye to open better and to improve vision.

The loss of V1 results in loss of sensation over the ipsilateral scalp, forehead, upper eyelid, cornea, nasal mucosa (frontal sinus), and nose. V2 loss results in loss of sensation from the ala, upper lip, maxillary dentition and gingiva, nasal mucosa (maxillary, ethmoid, and sphenoid sinuses), and hard and soft palate. Rehabilitation involves reassurance and avoidance of hot creams or emollients to prevent skin burns. The loss of sensation in the hard palate may put some people at risk for oral dysphagia because of the lack of palate sensation that triggers the tongue to propel a food bolus into the oropharynx.

The abducens (VI) nerve controls the lateral rectus and is particularly susceptible to injury during cavernous sinus surgery. It can be injured with tight packing of the cavernous sinus to control bleeding, despite the nerve being intact.[1] Initially, treatment entails observation with the use of refractive prism glasses. If the nerve is paralyzed, then transposition of superior and inferior rectus with Botulinum toxin injection in the ipsilateral medial rectus can help improve diplopia.[2]

Trigeminal Nerve (V3)

The third division of the trigeminal nerve has sensory and motor branches. The sensory branches include the buccal, inferior alveolar, lingual, auriculotemporal, and meningeal nerves. The last two cause skin sensory deficits and patients need to be instructed to be careful with grooming, including the use of hairdryers and curling irons because they can cause burns in the facial region because of lack of sensation. The buccal, inferior alveolar, and lingual nerves provide sensation to the inside of the mouth and can cause difficulty with swallowing. Hence, patients need to be prepared for this and may need swallowing therapy to allow for compensation. Grafting of these nerves, if possible, has been recommended.

The motor division of V3 supplies the following muscles: tensor veli palatini, tensor tympani, medial pterygoid, lateral pterygoid, temporalis, and masseter. Therapy for tensor veli palatini and tensor tympani loss is not needed because the function of palatal elevation (by tensor veli palatine) is compensated for by the levator veli palatini. The loss of tensor tympani results in reduced sound attenuation but is compensated for by the stapedius muscle. The rest of the muscles aid in mastication and if the contralateral muscles are intact, then the patient has minimum trismus or chewing problems. The issue of scarring and trismus can occur with extensive resection of the infratemporal fossa muscles. Such patients need to be placed on aggressive mandible physical therapy to keep the resultant fibrosis, and hence trismus, to a minimum. A stack of tongue depressors works well as self-directed physical therapy for patients. Temporalis and masseter wasting can occur by 1 year after sacrifice of V3 and this can be cosmetically corrected with silicone implants in the face and head.

Facial Nerve (VII)

The facial nerve provides movement to all the facial muscles of expression, the stapedius muscle, and the posterior belly of the digastric muscle. In addition, it provides taste to the anterior two thirds of the tongue by way of the chorda tympani nerve, and the palate by way of the pterygoid nerve and the greater superficial petrosal nerve. The facial nerve is saved in most cranial base procedures by way of facial nerve rerouting. In the event that the facial nerve is sacrificed, the resulting deficits are primarily due to motor dysfunction of the nerve. The most catastrophic of these events is the inability to close the eye and hence, risk for exposure keratitis and blindness. Lip droop can cause difficulty with swallowing and drooling because the oral commissure cannot form a complete seal to propel the food bolus posteriorly. Surgical rehabilitation methods to correct facial paralysis after cranial base surgery involve prostheses, neural anastomoses, and muscle flaps.

The most basic prosthetic device is a gold weight implant in the upper eyelid with the goal of allowing closure of the eyelid and hence, preventing exposure keratitis. A lateral tarsal strip procedure or tarsorrhaphy can also be performed to shorten the eyelid, correct the ectropion, and improve eye closure and lubrication.[3] Hypoglossal–facial nerve anastomosis has been described,[4] which allows the use of hypoglossal proximal fibers to help trigger the distal facial nerve branches. We have to be careful when considering hypoglossal–facial nerve transposition because many patients undergoing extensive skull base resections will have their vagus nerve injured, and a deficit in the hypoglossal nerve may be catastrophic for the patient's swallowing. The asymmetry of the mouth can be corrected with temporalis or masseter muscle transpositions, which act as dynamic facial slings.[5,6] If the trigeminal nerve has been sacrificed, then the neural supply to the temporalis and masseter muscle is compromised and these flaps will undergo atrophy with time. In general, for rehabilitation of the cranial nerve deficits, static slings for the face work more predictably. This procedure involves the placement of a sheet of acellular dermis or tensor fascia lata to pull the oral commissure superiorly in a more normal location, which allows for cosmetic improvement of the lips at rest. The gracilis free tissue transplant[7] has been a good alternative for restoring tone to the facial muscles. Overall, many options exist for the rehabilitation of the facial nerve. All procedures are aimed at improving cosmesis and function of the eye and oral commissure.

Vestibulocochlear Nerve (VIII)

The vestibulocochlear nerve provides sound and balance to the body. The auditory nerve transmits sound from the inner ear to the auditory cortex in the temporal lobe. If a translabyrinthine approach to the internal auditory canal is performed to remove a cerebellopontine angle tumor, then hearing and balance are destroyed. In most situations in which the patient undergoes extensive cranial base surgery, both branches of the VIII cranial nerve are affected. In this situation, the patient can undergo vestibular rehabilitation to improve balance. The patient may be able to be fitted with a contralateral routing of sound (CROS) hearing aid if he/she desires bilateral hearing and at least one ear has serviceable hearing.

Glossopharyngeal Nerve (IX)

The glossopharyngeal nerve has multiple functions that are related to swallowing. It has a visceral motor component that provides parasympathetic supply to the parotid gland. This supply reaches the parotid gland by way of the tympanic plexus in the middle ear and V3 by way of the otic ganglion. Injury to these branches may result in decreased salivary flow and hence, parotitis.

The general sensory component has afferent supply from the base of the tongue and pharynx, external ear, and external surface of the tympanic membrane. Damage to these fibers results in significant oropharyngeal dysphagia because of delay in oropharyngeal swallow. Isolated glossopharyngeal nerve deficit can be rehabilitated by aggressive swallow therapy, which focuses on trying to place the food bolus voluntarily on the sensate side of the pharynx.

The branchial motor component provides motor innervation to the stylopharyngeus muscle, which allows for elevation of the palate. Isolated loss to these fibers produces little difficulty in swallowing but when combined with the loss of the other fibers, severe dysphagia and velopharyngeal insufficiency can result.

Finally, the glossopharyngeal nerve carries visceral sensory information from the carotid body and sinus by way of the Hering nerve. Disruption of this nerve can result in carotid sinus syndrome. Ipsilateral loss usually does not cause problems with blood pressure, probably because of an intact system on the nonaffected side. If an individual has had contralateral surgery, then the possibility of carotid sinus syndrome should be entertained, with administration of beta-blockers and nitrates as needed.

Vagus Nerve (X)

The vagus nerve occupies the most central position in control of swallowing and the airway. Therefore, injury to the vagus nerve can have the most debilitating effects on the cranial base patient. The vagus nerve carries branchial motor, general sensory, visceral sensory, and visceral motor fibers.

The branchial motor fibers provide motor innervation by way of three distinct branches to the pharynx, palate, and larynx, except for the stylopharyngeus muscle (IX) and the tensor veli palatini (V3). The three branches are the pharyngeal branch, the external branch of the superior laryngeal nerve, and the recurrent laryngeal nerve. Injury to the pharyngeal branch results in paralysis of the ipsilateral palate and pharynx, leading to incomplete closure of the nasopharynx and hence, velopharyngeal insufficiency. The pharyngeal dysfunction responds well to swallowing therapy. Other modalities to improve velopharyngeal insufficiency include palatal obturators and palatal lift prostheses. Surgical approaches include pharyngeal augmentation (superiorly based) and pharyngoplasty. Another simple approach to treating velopharyngeal insufficiency is a palatal adhesion.[8] The palatal adhesion technique has become the procedure of choice in the authors' practice to correct hypernasality and nasal regurgitation, mainly because it does not require long flaps or alter the pharyngeal anatomy. They perform this procedure several months after the initial skull base surgery to allow for swallowing to stabilize and compensate with the swallowing therapy that the patient receives. The procedure is described later in this article, in the summary.

The paralysis of the constrictor muscles is more devastating than that of the palate. Normally, food would reach the oropharynx and then a downward constriction would push the food toward the hypopharynx while the larynx closes. With paralysis of the constrictors, the food is pushed toward the paralyzed side by the nonparalyzed side, resulting in bulging of the pharynx and delayed movement of the food bolus to the hypopharynx. Because the food stays in the hypopharynx and the larynx reopens, aspiration occurs. Treatment of this problem is centered on an intensive swallowing retraining program. Such a program emphasizes head positioning techniques that obliterate the paralyzed pharyngeal surface. In addition, avoidance of a tracheotomy can greatly help in swallowing therapy because it prevents the larynx from being "pegged" by a tube and allows for it to elevate normally (which is needed to prevent aspiration).

The external branch of the superior laryngeal nerve provides motor innervation to the cricothyroid muscle, which results in changes in vocal pitch. Because cranial base surgery usually results in high vagal transection or injury, the recurrent laryngeal nerve, which provides innervation to the intrinsic muscles of the larynx and the cricopharyngeus, can also be affected. The result is ipsilateral vocal cord paralysis and dysfunction of the cricopharyngeal muscle, which results in glottal incompetence with hoarseness and aspiration. In addition, the failure of cricopharyngeus relaxation also results in dysphagia and aspiration. Generally, a tracheotomy is performed in such cases for pulmonary toilet. In the authors' experience, most patients tolerate unilateral vocal cord paralysis well without tracheotomy. Initially, a Gelfoam medialization thyroplasty is performed (which can last up to 6 weeks) and then a permanent silastic medialization thyroplasty is performed at least 6 weeks after resection of the cranial base tumor. Silastic medialization thyroplasty with arytenoid adduction has been the authors' procedure of choice to address vocal fold paralysis in such patients. Cricopharyngeal myotomy can be performed and does allow for improved aspiration and assistance with swallowing therapy. The procedure for vocal fold medialization is described in the summary of this article.

The general sensory fibers of the vagus nerve provide sensation from the supraglottic larynx, lateral pharyngeal wall, external auditory canal, and tympanic membrane. The sensory fibers from the supraglottis form the superior laryngeal nerve and pass deep to the carotid arteries as they synapse to the inferior (nodose) ganglion. Loss of the superior laryngeal nerve can result in swallowing difficulties because of loss of sensation. Swallowing therapy is needed to rehabilitate this defect.

The visceral sensory fibers provide sensory and parasympathetic tone to the pharynx, larynx, esophagus, trachea, and thoracic and abdominal viscera down to the splenic flexure of the colon. Hence, unilateral loss of the vagus can result in reduced motility of the gastrointestinal tract, reduced tone of the lower esophageal sphincter, and delayed gastric emptying. These issues are dealt with by promotility pharmacologic agents, and a jejunal feeding tube may be needed in the early rehabilitation phase to prevent emesis. If bilateral vagal injuries occur, then a Nissen fundoplication may be needed to counter the esophageal sphincter dysfunction.

Spinal Accessory Nerve (XI)

The spinal accessory nerve is a motor nerve that innervates the sternocleidomastoid and trapezius muscles. It courses superficial to (70%), posterior to (27%), and through (3%) the internal jugular vein.[1] The resulting deficit is weakness in turning the head away from the operated side (sternocleidomastoid) and shoulder droop and pain with lateral rotation of the scapula (trapezius). In general, grafting of the spinal accessory nerve does not show much promise but such patients need to get enrolled in an aggressive physical therapy program for shoulder strengthening. This program may be needed indefinitely. Some patients undergo steroid injections for shoulder pain.

Hypoglossal Nerve (XII)

The hypoglossal nerve provides innervation to all intrinsic and extrinsic muscles of the tongue. It exits the skull base at the hypoglossal canal and as it curves laterally, it shares some fibers with the vagus nerve at the inferior (nodose) ganglion. Injury in this region can result in hypoglossal and vagal deficits, which can be morbid for the patient. The main issue with hypoglossal injury patients is that the food bolus cannot be propelled adequately during the oral phase of swallowing. Swallowing therapy is imperative in these situations.

SUMMARY

Cranial nerves play an important role in the functioning of an individual. Cranial base surgery can result in significant deficits that can be rehabilitated in various ways. Most patients will compensate well for their losses. Patients who have multiple cranial nerve injuries, especially of the glossopharyngeal, vagus, and hypoglossal nerves, can become swallowing cripples if not rehabilitated adequately. Such patients need to be followed with a multidisciplinary approach involving skull base surgery, laryngology, reconstructive surgery, and speech and swallowing therapy. Rehabilitation can take up to 1 year for a patient to reach a satisfactory functioning level.

Palatal Adhesion Technique

Preoperative assessment is accomplished by way of nasopharyngoscopy and swallow study. Under general anesthesia, the palate is exposed by way of a mouth gag. The paralyzed palate and posterior pharyngeal wall are injected with epinephrine for hemostasis. An incision is made through the palate along a palatal crease (**Fig. 1**). The posterior pharyngeal wall is viewed through this incision. An incision is made in the posterior pharyngeal wall down to the prevertebral fascia. Deep mattress sutures are placed to approximate the nasopharyngeal surface of the palate to the posterior pharyngeal wall (**Fig. 2**). The oral surface of the palate is closed and hence, a unilateral palatal adhesion is created.

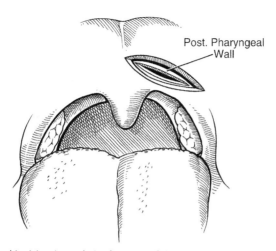

Fig. 1. A transpalatal incision is made in the area of the palatal crease that forms with normal palatal elevation and the posterior pharyngeal wall is viewed. (*From* Brackmann DE, Shelton C, Arriaga MA. Otologic surgery. 2nd edition. Philadelphia: WB Saunders; 2001. p. 493–502; with permission.)

Vocal Fold Medialization Technique

The goal for any vocal fold medialization in patients who have skull base surgery is to provide glottal competence, an effective cough for pulmonary toilet, and support and volume to voice.[1] Silastic medialization is performed under local anesthesia and is described well in the literature.[1,9–11] A midline horizontal incision is made over the mid-portion of the thyroid cartilage. The sternohyoid is detached from the hyoid bone and then the perichondrium over the thyroid cartilage is reflected posteriorly to leave it

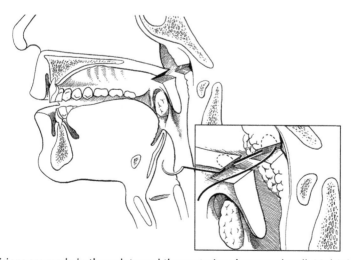

Fig. 2. Incisions are made in the palate and the posterior pharyngeal wall. Multiple mattress stitches are placed to complete the adhesion. (*From* Brackmann DE, Shelton C, Arriaga MA. Otologic surgery. 2nd edition. Philadelphia: WB Saunders; 2001. p. 493–502; with permission.)

pedicled posteriorly. In doing so, the thyrohyoid and sternothyroid muscles are elevated and the inferior edge of the thyroid cartilage is exposed. Then, a rectangular window is marked out so that the anterior edge of this lies 5 mm posterior to the anterior commissure in women and 7 mm posterior in men. The inferior edge of the window is created so a 3-mm strut of cartilage is left inferiorly. A drill is then used to drill out this cartilage window. The inner perichondrium is then elevated in all directions except anteriorly. The perichondrium is incised. The depth gauge is used to medialize the vocal cord, and voice quality is assessed. Then, using these dimensions, the silastic block is carved, with the point of maximum medialization at the lower border of the window. The block is inserted in the window and secured with 4-0 Prolene stitches.

REFERENCES

1. Netterville JL, Sullivan CA. Rehabilitation of lower cranial nerve deficits after neurotologic skull base surgery. In: Brackmann, et al, Otologic surgery. 48. 2nd edition. WB Saunders; 2001. p. 493–502.
2. Rosenbaum AL, Kushyner B. Vertical rectus muscle transposition and botulinum toxin after abducens nerve palsy. Arch Ophthalmol 1989;107:820–3.
3. Becker FF. Lateral tarsal strip procedure for the correction of paralytic ectropion. Laryngoscope 1982;92(4):382–4.
4. Arai H, Sato K, Yanai A. Hemihypoglossal-facial nerve anastomosis in treating unilateral facial palsy after acoustic neurinoma resection. J Neurosurg 1995;82(1): 51–4.
5. Cheney ML, McKenna MJ, Megerian CA, et al. Early temporalis muscle transposition for the management of facial paralysis. Laryngoscope 1995;105:993–1000.
6. Burgess LPA, Goode RL. Total facial paralysis. In: Burgess LPA, Goode RL, editors. Reanimation of the paralyzed face. New York: Thieme Medical Publishers; 1994. p. 11–26.
7. Chuang DC, Mardini S, Lin SH, et al. Free proximal gracilis muscle and its skin paddle compound flap transplantation for complex facial paralysis. Plast Reconstr Surg 2004;113(1):126–32 [discussion: 133–5].
8. Netterville JL, Vrabec JT. Unilateral palatal adhesion for paralysis after high vagal injury. Arch Otolaryngol Head Neck Surg 1994;120:218–21.
9. Netterville JL, Jackson CG, Civantos FJ. Thyroplasty in the functional rehabilitation of neurotologic skull base surgery patients. Am J Otol 1993;14:460–4.
10. Netterville JL, Stone RE, Lukens LS, et al. Silastic medialization and arytenoid adduction: the Vanderbilt experience - a review of 116 phonosurgical procedures. Ann Otol Rhinol Laryngol 1993;102:413–24.
11. Wanamaker JR, Netterville JL, Ossoff RH. Phonosurgery: silastic medialization for unilateral vocal fold paralysis. Operative Techniques in Otolaryngology Head and Neck Surgery 1993;4:207.

Palliative Aspects of Recurrent Respiratory Papillomatosis

Kaalan Johnson, MD[a], Craig Derkay, MD[a,b],*

KEYWORDS

- Recurrent respiratory papillomatosis • Human papillomavirus
- HPV vaccine

Recurrent respiratory papillomatosis (RRP) is a disorder characterized by the presence within the larynx, trachea, and sometimes even lungs of benign papillomata that have a tendency to grow causing airway obstruction and to recur after surgical removal. The airway obstruction that is so often present with RRP can be severe and life-threatening such that these patients usually require vigilant monitoring and prompt endoscopic surgical treatment as soon as the airway begins to be compromised. The papillomata seen in RRP are caused by human papillomavirus (HPV). RRP has a bimodal age of onset with juvenile-onset RRP (JORRP) behaving somewhat differently than adult-onset RRP (AORRP). The clinical course of RRP is also highly variable. Some more fortunate patients experience spontaneous regression so that they only need a few endoscopic procedures throughout their lifetime and seem to be cured of the disease, even though they still harbor the virus at a cellular level. Other patients who have relentlessly recurring and aggressive papillomata lead difficult lives fraught with hundreds of operations and potentially the ominous spectrum of disease progression, which may include pulmonary lesions or, even worse, the transformation from RRP to squamous cell carcinoma. Maintaining a unique approach to these patients in family interactions, office protocols, and operative interventions results in improved outcomes and patient satisfaction in this frequently devastating disease.

ETIOLOGY AND EPIDEMIOLOGY
Virology of Human Papillomavirus

RRP was first confirmed to contain HPV DNA in 1980 by Quick and coworkers,[1,2] with further characterization and typing by Gissmann and coworkers[3] and Mounts and

[a] Department of Otolaryngology – Head and Neck Surgery, Eastern Virginia Medical School, Norfolk, VA, USA
[b] Department of Pediatrics, Eastern Virginia Medical School, Norfolk, VA, USA
* Corresponding author. Children's Hospital of the King's Daughters, 601 Children's Lane, Norfolk, VA 23507.
E-mail address: craig.derkay@chkd.org (C. Derkay).

Otolaryngol Clin N Am 42 (2009) 57–70
doi:10.1016/j.otc.2008.09.007
0030-6665/08/$ – see front matter © 2009 Elsevier Inc. All rights reserved.

coworkers[4] in 1982, although it had been the presumed etiology for decades. HPV is an icosahedral (20-sided) DNA capsid virus that is categorized based on genetic homology into greater than 180 identified genotypes, which correspond to different tissue preferences and clinical manifestations.[5] HPV types 6 and 11 account for the most cases of RRP. HPV-11 occurs most commonly (52%–62% of isolates) and runs the most aggressive clinical course, followed by HPV-6 (24%–48%).[5-7] HPV types 16, 18, 31, and 33 have also rarely been reported in RRP.[8]

Malignant transformation occurs in cervical cancers most commonly with HPV types 16 and 18, with HPV-6 and -11 described as low-risk and HPV-31 and -33 intermediate-risk.[9] In RRP this has generally been reported in adults with other risk factors, such as tobacco use or exposure to radiation, but also occurs in children who commonly have prolonged, extensive disease with distal spread.[10] The etiology of transformation is thought by some authors to follow a gradual molecular transformation. In one example this involved integration of HPV-11 DNA into the host genome in malignant tissue samples and mutation of the p53 proto-oncogene.[11] In their largest series of nine patients, Reidy and colleagues[12] found HPV-11 to be present in all evaluable malignant samples, and RNA assays showed evidence of HPV integration in three of seven sufficient samples. No evaluation of p53 status was performed in this study. In five sufficient samples from seven patients with malignant transformation, Go and colleagues[13] agreed with the consistent expression of HPV-11 in malignancy, and found p53 expression to be variable, but was not able to demonstrate a progressive histologic appearance in serial samples. The palliative treatment of the common clinical course of recurrent airway obstruction and hoarseness in RRP is redirected when malignant transformation occurs with conventional head and neck cancer treatment superseding original treatment goals. Most squamous cell carcinomas arising with a history of RRP are well-differentiated, and when occurring in the lung, these seem to have a refractory clinical course.[13]

Transmission

Transmission of RRP classically occurs in the vaginally delivered first-born child of a teenage mother of low socioeconomic status. This has been reported in 30% to 75% of JORRP cases, although recent data have questioned the association of socioeconomic status and disease severity.[14] The classic explanation for AORRP transmission occurs in patients with multiple oral sexual partners. D'Souza and colleagues[15] in a recent case-control study published in the *New England Journal of Medicine* found a significant association between lifetime vaginal-sex and oral-sex partners and oropharyngeal squamous cell carcinomas. HPV-16 infection produced an odds ratio of 33.6 ($P<.05$) for the development of squamous cell carcinomas in those studied. Neither of these theories is sufficient, however, to explain onset of disease in patients without these exposures or why most patients with these exposures do not develop RRP. Shah and colleagues[16] has suggested that one in several hundred children born to a mother with active HPV condylomata develops RRP. HPV prevalence in the United States is alarmingly high with 60% of women of childbearing age (80 million) found to be HPV antibody positive but DNA negative; 10% (14 million) DNA positive; and 1% with active genital papillomas. Condylomata have been found in pregnant women at a rate of 1.5% to 5%.[8] With 3.6 million annual births in the United States, these values do not account for the observed RRP incidence of 4.3 per 100,000 children.[17] Development of clinical RRP is clearly a multifactorial process that is still poorly understood. Elective cesarean section delivery does not prevent every case of RRP, and is not routinely indicated at this time for at-risk mothers, although this decision warrants discussion with an individual's birth care provider.[18]

CLINICAL FEATURES
Patient Assessment

History
JORRP (ordinarily defined as an age of diagnosis before 12 years) commonly presents between 2 and 4 years of age with hoarseness, which may progress over weeks or months to stridor (inspiratory early, progressing to biphasic); increased work of breathing; and complete airway obstruction if not addressed. The diagnosis is typically confirmed around 1 year after initial development of symptoms. Less common presenting symptoms include chronic cough, recurrent pneumonia, dysphagia, failure to thrive, dyspnea, or acute life-threatening events. AORRP peaks between ages 20 and 40 years of age with a slight male predilection and generally a slightly more benign clinical course than JORRP. Characterizing the time course of progression and risk factors may distinguish RRP from other airway pathology, such as subglottic stenosis, vocal cord paralysis, tracheomalacia, laryngomalacia, or subglottic hemangiomas or cysts. Voice use and vocal hygiene and progression may be useful to differentiate RRP from vocal nodules, which is the most common cause of hoarseness in children (RRP is second). Lastly, a complete medical, family, and social history is essential, including parental history of genital papilloma disease.[8,10]

Physical examination
All patients should be assessed at presentation with a complete age-appropriate head and neck examination, specifically including a close observation of general appearance and auscultation of the upper airway. Patients with signs of air-hunger including neck extension, leaning forward with forearm support of the upper body (the tripod position), nasal flaring, drooling, use of accessory muscles of respiration, or cyanosis may not warrant any further evaluation before proceeding directly to the emergency department or the operating room. Auscultation is performed in the stable patient over the lower lung fields, trachea, larynx, and pharynx, using the open end of the stethoscope tube if necessary in patients with a small or short neck. Correlating laryngeal auscultation with operative endoscopy may provide very detailed information regarding the airway status in follow-up patients.

A complete office evaluation also generally includes a flexible fiberoptic examination of the upper airway if equipment and patient cooperation and stability allow. After application of a topical decongestant (with a topical anesthetic in larger children or adults) the nasopharynx, oropharynx, hypopharynx, larynx, and subglottis are sequentially evaluated dynamically. Care should be taken closely to examine the squamocolumnar junctions of the airway (ie, the limen nasi, soft palate, ventricle, and the undersurface of the true vocal folds) because these transition zones have been shown to have a predilection for RRP manifestation.[8] In most cases this examination provides the clinician with diagnostic confirmation of RRP (and most other entities in the differential diagnosis). More importantly, it provides essential prognostic information regarding the location, severity, and acuity of disease involvement and dictates timing of follow-up or operative intervention.

Airway endoscopy
The next step in most cases is endoscopy in the operating room. If emergent or urgent, this may be arranged as soon as the operating room can be made ready with supportive care in the emergency department until that time. If stable, the procedure may be scheduled to occur days or weeks in the future depending on the location, extent of disease, and expected progression. Informed consent is obtained detailing the risks of bleeding complications, infections, scarring, or stenotic complications; likely

need for further procedures; possible tracheotomy; anesthesia complications; and airway compromise or death. Once in the operating room, anesthesia is induced and the airway is evaluated by the surgeon generally using a Parsons laryngoscope and zero-degree telescope with photographs taken before any intervention for diagnostic and staging purposes (**Fig. 1**). Once the diagnosis is confirmed and documented, debridement is performed as indicated.

Staging and severity

Several methods of staging RRP have been proposed that vary in complexity and usefulness. The goals of each are to provide a standardization of RRP evaluation and improve effectiveness in communication between otolaryngologists, clinical monitoring, and research protocol performance. One of the most popular and the authors' preferred method for staging was developed out of a committee of the American Society of Pediatric Otolaryngology (ASPO) in 1998. It has been included in a software package developed at the University of Washington (Seattle) and licensed to ASPO to ease data input and tracking for patients with RRP.[19] This scheme identifies a 0- to 86-point score with 4 clinical and 25 anatomic components (**Fig. 2**). It has been shown to have good reliability between surgeon raters[20] and good prognostic value for some elements to predict decreased surgical interval.[21]

SURGICAL MANAGEMENT
Anesthetic Techniques

The intricacies of anesthetic management are just as important as the surgical intervention in the complicated and dangerous airways of RRP patients. Using an experienced anesthesia team and communicating early and clearly are crucial to the safe management of this disease. In practices that had experienced an RRP-related death, anesthesia-related complications were the second most common cause accounting for 7 (22.6%) of 31 deaths reported in an ASPO survey.[22]

Traditional techniques for airway management used laser-safe endotracheal tubes. Reports have now cast suspicion on increased airway instrumentation contributing to distal spread of disease (including tracheotomy as discussed later). The most preferred methods of anesthesia among current members of ASPO are spontaneous or intermittent apneic ventilation (63.5% of respondents in a recent survey), with 24.3% using jet ventilation and 9.6% laser-safe endotracheal tubes.[22]

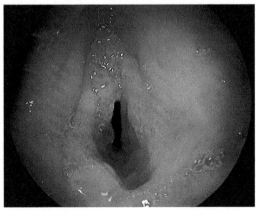

Fig. 1. Endoscopic photograph of laryngeal recurrent respiratory papillomatosis.

Staging assessment sheet.[4]

STAGING ASSESSMENT FOR RECURRENT LARYNGEAL PAPILLOMATOSIS

PATIENT INITIALS:____   DATE OF SURGERY:____   SURGEON:____
PATIENT ID #:____   INSTITUTION:____

1. How long since the last papilloma surgery? ____days, ____weeks, ____months, ____years, ____don't know, ____1st surgery

2. Counting today's surgery, how many papilloma surgeries in the past 12 months? ____

3. Describe the patient's voice today: ____aphonic, ____ abnormal, ____normal , ____other

4. Describe the patient's stridor today: ____absent, ____present with activity, ____present at rest, ____don't know

5. Describe the urgency of today's intervention: ____scheduled, ____urgent, ____emergent

FOR EACH SITE, SCORE AS: 0 = none, 1 = surface lesion, 2 = raised lesion, 3 = bulky lesion

LARYNX
    Epiglottis
    Lingual surface_____Laryngeal surface_____
    Aryepiglottic folds: Right____ Left____
    False vocal cords: Right____ Left____
    True vocal cords: Right____ Left____
    Arytenoids: Right____ Left____
    Anterior commisure_____   Posterior commisure_____
    Subglottis _____

TRACHEA:
    Upper one-third _____
    Middle one-third_____
    Lower one-third_____
    Bronchi: Right _____   Left_____
    Tracheotomy stoma_____

OTHER:
    Nose _____
    Palate _____
    Pharynx _____
    Esophagus_____
    Lungs _____
    Other _____

TOTAL SCORE ALL SITES:_____

Fig. 2. Coltrera-Derkay staging and severity scheme. (*From* Derkay CS, Malis DJ, Zalzal G, et al. A staging system for assessing severity of disease and response to therapy in recurrent respiratory papillomatosis. Laryngoscope 1998;108:935–7; with permission.)

Classic Surgical Techniques

In the absence of any medically curative treatment, surgical resection of obstructing papillomatous lesions has been the mainstay of palliative treatment for RRP. The goals of surgery are to ensure an adequate airway and functional voice for the greatest possible period before papillomas recur without damaging any healthy underlying tissue that would predispose the patient to long-term complications of scarring, stenosis, and dysphonia.

Placement of a tracheotomy tube is the oldest treatment modality for RRP disease. Although generally avoided today, it is occasionally still necessary for advanced disease or stenotic complications.[23] Concern has been raised regarding the role of tracheotomy tubes in potentiating distal spread of RRP.[24] Cole and colleagues[25] reviewed their experience with 12 tracheotomized patients with RRP, of whom six developed distal spread of disease. They found distal spread to associate with subglottic disease at the time of tracheotomy, and this was observed to progress from involvement of stomal mucosa to the mid-trachea in an average of 10 weeks. Tracheotomy introduces a novel squamocolumnar junction into the airway with a predilection for RRP involvement as discussed previously.[8] Shapiro and colleagues[26] questioned the etiology of distal spread by noting that in 13 of 35 patients reviewed who required tracheotomy, presentation occurred at an earlier age with more advanced disease often involving the distal airway. Distal spread occurred in 50% but was generally limited to the tracheotomy site. The review by Chen and Liu,[27] however, continued to demonstrate the strong association between tracheotomy and distal disease (80.9%). In the palliative treatment of RRP, consideration of tracheotomy placement is one of the most important surgical decision points. Most authors would agree that tracheotomy is necessary in the worst obstructive and most rapidly refractory cases of RRP, and generally still have good outcomes. But this still should be avoided when the disease is able to be managed transorally.[8,10,28]

Microsurgical excision was the earliest transoral management option for RRP and is still a preferred treatment in AORRP with limited involvement. Standard microlaryngeal instruments and techniques may be used completely to excise laryngeal papillomata with good voice results, and in one recent series complete remission was observed in 2-year follow-up of six primary AORRP patients.[29] This treatment is not as effective in recurrent or extensive disease, and may result in web formation or scarring of the superficial layer of the lamina propria.[29,30]

Emerging Techniques

The carbon dioxide (CO_2) laser has been a mainstay of treatment for RRP since its introduction to endolaryngeal surgery in the 1970s. Laser energy is absorbed by water in the tissues resulting in ablation, and when coupled with an operating microscope, may result in precise, hemostatic vaporization of papillomas with minimal damage to underlying normal tissues. Newer ultrapulsed laser models with a micromanipulator allow for less surrounding tissue destruction with beam-shaping capabilities to form a dot, line, circle, or arc to increase even further the precision of tissue ablation. Fiber delivery systems are also being developed for the CO_2 laser (Omniguide, Cambridge, Massachusetts), which have shown good cutting efficacy and healing characteristics in early studies[31] and may provide additional flexibility for ablating papilloma disease in difficult locations endoscopically.

The microdebrider is a device that uses suction and rotating cold blade excision precisely to remove papillomas. The 4-mm laryngeal Skimmer blade (Medtronic, Jacksonville, Florida) has been designed for microlaryngeal use. With its slightly angulated tip, it allows mobile papilloma tissue to be drawn by the suction into the cutting blade and leaves firmer underlying native tissues undisturbed. A prospective comparison found that use of the microdebrider resulted in equivalent postoperative pain with greater improvements in voice quality, shorter procedure times, and a lower overall procedure cost compared with the CO_2 laser.[32] Use of the microdebrider has recently supplanted the CO_2 laser (previously favored by 92% of respondents)[17] as the most popular device for excision of papillomas in JORRP according to a survey of ASPO members.[22]

Recent years have seen an increase in the use of angiolytic lasers for treatment of RRP. These include the 585-nm pulsed dye laser and the 532-nm pulsed potassium-titanyl-phosphate laser, which are absorbed selectively by hemoglobin, causing selective tissue ablation in the highly vascular papilloma lesions.

In a series of 47 patients treated with office-based pulsed dye laser with a mean 13.2-month follow-up, 60% of 117 procedures were performed for RRP with good effect. Thirty percent of cases had anterior commissure involvement, and no incidences of scarring or webs were reported (pulsed dye laser is actually indicated as a treatment for hypertrophic scarring). No complications were noted in RRP patients, with only one complication in the series noted in a patient with Reinke's edema who developed worsening airway edema and required admission for observation and corticosteroid therapy.[33]

The 532-nm pulsed potassium-titanyl-phosphate laser therapy has been used for in-office and general anesthetic management of AORRP. In a pilot study by Burns and colleagues[30] of 55 procedures in 37 patients with RRP, disease regression and improvement in subjective dysphonia were noted in all patients who had appropriate follow-up with 80% showing disease regression of 90% or more. Ninety-three percent of the patients had anterior commissure disease, and no occurrence of synechiae or web formation was found in near-term follow-up (defined as 1–3 months). This laser has been approved by the Food and Drug Administration (FDA) for ablation of vascular lesions of the upper airway including papillomas. Further basic science and clinical work is ongoing for operating room and in-office application of this therapeutic option.[30,34]

Angiolytic lasers are an exciting advancement with documented efficacy.[34,35] In adults or tolerant older children these lasers may be used for in-office management of RRP with significant advantages in cost and patient convenience. This technology may change the face of adult management of RRP in coming years as financial accessibility increases.

MEDICAL MANAGEMENT
Antiviral Therapy

Traditional antiviral medications including acyclovir (Zovirax) and ribavirin (Rebetol, Virazole, Copegas) have been attempted as adjuvant therapy in RRP. Ribavirin is used to treat infants with respiratory syncytial virus, and has shown an increased surgical interval in ribavirin-treated patients in an uncontrolled trial of four patients.[36] Acyclovir is thought to improve results in RRP by decreasing cellular coinfection by other viruses,[37] and has been used in three small uncontrolled trials with positive results.[38]

Most trials of adjuvant therapy have used cidofovir (Vistide) by intralesional injection or intravenous administration. Cidofovir is a nucleoside analogue with FDA approval for treating cytomegalovirus retinitis in HIV and AIDS patients but is seldom used for this indication now because of significant nephrotoxicity and availability of less toxic alternatives. Fourteen studies have looked at efficacy of intralesional cidofovir with case series generally demonstrating favorable results with low numbers of nonresponders.[38] One small historical case-control study by Mandell and colleagues[39] in 2004 compared four children treated with surgical debulking and intralesional cidofovir every 2 months until remission with three severity-matched controls who only received surgeries as indicated for their disease. Significantly improved severity scores were achieved in cidofovir-treated versus control patients, although the study was weakened by lack of placebo, randomization, blinding, and small sample size. Concerns have also been raised regarding the carcinogenic potential of cidofovir when mammary adenocarcinomas occurred in rats at one twenty-fifth the recommended human dose. For this reason the Task Force on RRP has recommended limiting usage of adjuvant cidofovir to dosages of less than 5 mg/kg, and to only severe recalcitrant cases (ie, those requiring greater than three surgical procedures per year, worsening airway compromise, or severely impaired communication, or those otherwise considered candidates for tracheotomy).[40] Intravenous cidofovir showed positive effects in three reports of extremely severe cases and should be reserved for only these situations.[38]

Multiple other adjuvant therapies have been tried and are generally believed to have some benefit, but limitations in data preclude significant clinical conclusions about indole 3-carbinol; retinoids; celecoxib (Celebrex); retinoids; and photodynamic therapy. Interferon-α has shown clinical benefit, although it has a rebound effect and significant toxicity.[38,41]

Extraesophageal Reflux

Extraesophageal reflux has been implicated as a negative prognostic indicator in severe RRP. McKenna and Brodsky[42] reviewed four children in whom reflux seemed to worsen RRP disease burden and antireflux therapy was subsequently associated with improvement. In three out of the four patients a temporary lapse in compliance with reflux therapy triggered worsening of their RRP. Pignatari and colleagues[43] also demonstrated proximal reflux on pH probes in 9 of 10 patients with RRP, with 5 of 10 believed to be pathologic reflux. Fifteen percent of ASPO members routinely prescribe antireflux medication and give reflux precautions in patients with RRP based on data demonstrating reduced scarring and web formation in RRP patients treated prophylactically for reflux.[22]

OTHER THERAPIES
Immunotherapy

Heat shock protein E7 is the fusion protein of recombinant heat shock protein 65 from *Mycobacterium bovis* and the E7 protein from HPV-16. Subcutaneous administration of three doses of heat shock protein E7 after debulking surgery showed significant lengthening of surgical intervals, especially in female patients.[44] This product is not currently commercially available but may have some clinical use in the future. Immunologic modification is clearly central to the future prevention and possible eradication of RRP (see later) and may play an important role in therapy for RRP. With the quadrivalent HPV recombinant vaccine (Gardisil) now commercially available, clinical trials are under development to examine the therapeutic in addition to the preventative possibilities of this vaccine in RRP (Farrel Buchinsky, personal communication, 2007).

PREVENTION
Birth Considerations

Prolonged exposure to active papillomatous lesions during a primagravid birth is thought to increase risk of development of RRP, although this does not completely explain the pathogenesis of contraction (as discussed previously). All pregnant women should be evaluated for HPV infection and treated when indicated, but prophylactic cesarean section delivery is controversial.[45]

Cesarean section delivery does not prevent development of RRP in every case, but some have argued that because of the extremely high cost of RRP cases (with a prevalence of 4.3 in children and 1.8 in adults per 100,000 population, annual costs for RRP still exceed $150 million in health care dollars annually and 15,000 procedures),[17] it is less of a medical financial burden to perform elective cesarean section deliveries on all high-risk pregnancies.[18] This is not a current recommendation of the American College of Obstetrics and Gynecology and should be approached individually with each woman and her obstetrician.

Socioeconomic status has long been considered a risk factor for development of RRP.[8] Socioeconomic status was not found to correlate with disease severity in a recent Canadian study, but national data collection is underway.[14]

Recurrent Respiratory Papillomatosis Registry and Task Force

In January 1997, the Centers for Disease Control and Prevention initiated a registry of patients with RRP to include 600 patients across 20 institutions. The goals of the registry were to promote standardization of patient tracking, outcomes analysis, and protocol development further to elucidate therapeutic objectives and outcomes in this rare and devastating disease. The RRP Task Force was developed through coordination by ASPO as a committee of principal investigators at each registry institution, members of the adult RRP research community, and representatives from advocacy groups. The Task Force meets twice yearly to further research initiatives for this disease.[41] Several publications and opinions have emerged from this group since that time,[17,40,44,46] and ongoing work regarding the vaccine for RRP is being coordinated through its efforts.

Human Papillomavirus Vaccines

Work began in 1991 on creating a vaccine against the most common and pathogenic strains of HPV at multiple institutions. Virus-like particles are created from self-assembled HPV L1 proteins, which have antigenic properties but are not virulent. Virus-like particles were developed at universities in Rochester, Queensland, and at the National Cancer Institute, but the patent on virus-like particles is currently held after much conflict by Georgetown University for their development of the "background science" behind this discovery.[47] Two vaccines have currently been developed and studied and the quadrivalent HPV recombinant vaccine, which has shown efficacy against HPV-16 and -18 and additionally HPV-6 and -11, has received FDA approval for implementation among school-aged girls. Interest is growing even outside of otolaryngology about potential ancillary effects of HPV vaccination on RRP reduction or eradication, which will be enthusiastically tracked over the next few decades after vaccine introduction.[48] Epidemiologic modeling analyses of vaccine implementation anticipate reduced long-term cervical cancer incidence and cost-effectiveness of vaccination with regard to cervical cancer, without even considering the potential cost benefits of a reduced incidence of cancers of the vagina, vulva, anus, penis, and head and neck, or RRP.[49] Points of interest for future debates include administration of the vaccine to boys, neonatal administration to prevent childhood development of RRP, and therapeutic use of the vaccine in developed cases of RRP in attempts at immune-modulated regression of disease.

PALLIATIVE AND RECALCITRANT CARE
Therapeutic Considerations

The most important therapeutic considerations, which are dictated by the chronicity and palliative nature of RRP, involve the conservative nature of interventions. The central aims of surgical procedures are always to remove the obstructing lesions as completely as possible to maximize the surgical interval and phonatory outcomes while never violating normal tissue. Treating reflux is also important to avoid long-term soft tissue complications. Papillomas grow back to be removed another day until remission is attained, but overzealous resection may result in webbing or stenosis, which is very difficult to treat and frequently life-long. Side effect profiles and associated risks of malignant transformation also require extremely conservative application of adjuvant medical therapies to only the most severely affected individuals.

Office Management

Office protocols must be uniquely structured to handle RRP patients. Especially in JORRP patients, every staff member from the front office personnel to the head nurse and physicians must be very clear that if a patient or parent of a child with RRP calls with a respiratory concern, they need to be triaged by an experienced nurse or a physician and often evaluated in the office or operating room within hours or days of the contact. Parents of children with RRP develop an intimate familiarity with the progression of their child's disease, and begin to recognize how much time remains before their child's acuity worsens. In severe cases, postoperative follow-up or scheduled office appointments are often unnecessary, and patients may proceed directly to the operating room when they or their parents determine that they are in need of surgery. This may range from 0.2 to 19.3 procedures per year, but the average child with active RRP requires 4.4 procedures (ie, an operative procedure every 2–3 months).[46] This has a tremendously burdensome effect on these patients and families, which must be kept in consideration not just by the treating physicians but also by the remainder of the office and operating room staff.

Psychosocial Considerations

Quality of life has been recently looked at in more detail in this disease. Hill and colleagues[50] in London evaluated 26 adult patients by a postal survey using two methods of quality-of-life analysis. They found good correlation between disease severity as diagnosed clinically and detrimental effect on quality of life, especially on social functioning domains. Lindman and colleagues[51] from the University of Alabama recently evaluated subjective (voice-related quality-of-life questionnaire), objective (speech therapist graded GRBAS [Grade of hoarseness, Roughness, Breathiness, Asthenia, and Strain]), and acoustic analysis to determine quality of life in children with quiescent RRP. Four children with no active disease for 12 months were age and gender matched to four controls without RRP. Subjective measures showed no perception of a functional difference between groups, but blinded speech pathology evaluations showed significantly more hoarse, breathy, and rough voices in patients with acoustic analyses confirming lower fundamental frequencies, and higher relative average perturbations. A follow-up study in patients with active disease used a validated[52] pediatric instrument, the PedsQL 4.0, to compare 22 patients with RRP with validated normals for healthy children and children with a chronic illness. All domains showed significantly lower health-related quality of life in RRP compared with healthy children, and were generally similar to children with other chronic illnesses. Children with RRP, however, had even worse scores in psychosocial health and school functioning domains than chronic illness normals.[53]

These realities will be further studied in coming years, but should be taken into account when dealing with these children in the clinic and especially operating room settings. Procedures become routine and commonplace to these children, and great care should be taken to make this painful process as easy as possible for the child, for their own sake and for the sake of the health care providers who care for the child in the future.

Family Dynamics

Families of children or patients with RRP adapt in a variety of ways to their situation. Some are extremely involved, sensitive, and informed about their loved-one's condition and make every effort to assist and support. Others do obligatory duties and little else. Rarely, family members are completely apathetic or even harsh to the patient. Health care providers need to be very sensitive to the attitudes of not only the patient but their family support structure. The attentiveness of the family members, especially for young children, may be as important as the patient's disease process in predicting outcomes and acuity. Special considerations, such as regularly scheduled appointments or social worker interventions, may be appropriate depending on the competence, awareness, and involvement of the family support network.

SUMMARY

RRP is a benign viral infectious disease of the upper aerodigestive tract that can result in life-threatening airway compromise and frequently requires long-long palliative treatment. Complete evaluation of the patients with office endoscopy and careful attention to anatomic site involvement, acuity, and patient-family dependability help in structuring therapeutic plans that are safe and effective for patients with this condition. Operative endoscopy and treatment should be scheduled early and regularly based on these considerations and always undertaken with great care in concert with a qualified anesthesia team.

Operative management is the mainstay of current RRP treatment, and consists of debridement of obstructive papillomatous lesions while carefully preserving underlying normal tissue to avoid stenotic or dysphonic complications. Microdebrider followed by CO_2 laser are the mainstays of treatment; emerging angiolytic laser techniques are gaining popularity especially in adult, in-office settings; and tracheotomy should be reserved for only the most severe cases. Adjuvant therapy with cidofovir is also reserved only for severe cases (generally requiring four or more procedures per year) because of its carcinogenic potential and paucity of high-level supportive data.

The quadrivalent Gardisil vaccine targets HPV-6, -11, -16, and -18, and is currently recommended for all school-aged girls. With more widespread use including administration to males, this vaccine has the potential not only to decrease cervical cancer incidence but potentially to eradicate RRP in the future. Therapeutic use of the vaccine is under study as a potential future adjuvant therapy for existing disease.

Psychosocial, family dynamic, and quality-of-life issues are paramount to the appropriate and safe palliative management of this difficult and frequently devastating disease and should always be considered by the entire care team in the therapeutic approach to these unique patients.

REFERENCES

1. Quick CA, Watts SL, Krzyzek RA, et al. Relationship between condylomata and laryngeal papillomata: clinical and molecular virological evidence. Ann Otol Rhinol Laryngol 1980;89(5 Pt 1):467–71.
2. Bauman NM, Smith RJ. Recurrent respiratory papillomatosis. Pediatr Clin North Am 1996;43(6):1385–401.
3. Gissmann L, Diehl V, Schultz-Coulon HJ, et al. Molecular cloning and characterization of human papilloma virus DNA derived from a laryngeal papilloma. J Virol 1982;44(1):393–400.

4. Mounts P, Shah KV, Kashima H. Viral etiology of juvenile- and adult-onset squamous papilloma of the larynx. Proc Natl Acad Sci U S A 1982;79(17):5425–9.

5. Draganov P, Todorov S, Todorov I, et al. Identification of HPV DNA in patients with juvenile-onset recurrent respiratory papillomatosis using SYBR Green real-time PCR. Int J Pediatr Otorhinolaryngol 2006;70(3):469–73.

6. Wiatrak BJ, Wiatrak DW, Broker TR, et al. Recurrent respiratory papillomatosis: a longitudinal study comparing severity associated with human papilloma viral types 6 and 11 and other risk factors in a large pediatric population. Laryngoscope 2004;114(11 Pt 2 Suppl 104):1–23.

7. Rabah R, Lancaster WD, Thomas R, et al. Human papillomavirus-11-associated recurrent respiratory papillomatosis is more aggressive than human papillomavirus-6-associated disease. Pediatr Dev Pathol 2001;4(1):68–72.

8. Derkay CS, Darrow DH. Recurrent respiratory papillomatosis. Ann Otol Rhinol Laryngol 2006;115(1):1–11.

9. Rimell F, Maisel R, Dayton V. In situ hybridization and laryngeal papillomas. Ann Otol Rhinol Laryngol 1992;101(2 Pt 1):119–26.

10. Stamataki S, Nikolopoulos TP, Korres S, et al. Juvenile recurrent respiratory papillomatosis: still a mystery disease with difficult management. Head Neck 2007;29(2):155–62.

11. Rady PL, Schnadig VJ, Weiss RL, et al. Malignant transformation of recurrent respiratory papillomatosis associated with integrated human papillomavirus type 11 DNA and mutation of p53. Laryngoscope 1998;108(5):735–40.

12. Reidy PM, Dedo HH, Rabah R, et al. Integration of human papillomavirus type 11 in recurrent respiratory papilloma-associated cancer. Laryngoscope 2004; 114(11):1906–9.

13. Go C, Schwartz MR, Donovan DT. Molecular transformation of recurrent respiratory papillomatosis: viral typing and p53 overexpression. Ann Otol Rhinol Laryngol 2003;112(4):298–302.

14. Leung R, Hawkes M, Campisi P. Severity of juvenile onset recurrent respiratory papillomatosis is not associated with socioeconomic status in a setting of universal health care. Int J Pediatr Otorhinolaryngol 2007;71(6):965–72.

15. D'Souza G, Kreimer AR, Viscidi R, et al. Case-control study of human papillomavirus and oropharyngeal cancer. N Engl J Med 2007;356(19):1944–56.

16. Shah K, Kashima H, Polk BF, et al. Rarity of cesarean delivery in cases of juvenile-onset respiratory papillomatosis. Obstet Gynecol 1986;68(6):795–9.

17. Derkay CS. Task force on recurrent respiratory papillomas: a preliminary report. Arch Otolaryngol Head Neck Surg 1995;121(12):1386–91.

18. Bishai D, Kashima H, Shah K. The cost of juvenile-onset recurrent respiratory papillomatosis. Arch Otolaryngol Head Neck Surg 2000;126(8):935–9.

19. Derkay CS, Malis DJ, Zalzal G, et al. A staging system for assessing severity of disease and response to therapy in recurrent respiratory papillomatosis. Laryngoscope 1998;108(6):935–7.

20. Hester RP, Derkay CS, Burke BL, et al. Reliability of a staging assessment system for recurrent respiratory papillomatosis. Int J Pediatr Otorhinolaryngol 2003;67(5): 505–9.

21. Derkay CS, Hester RP, Burke B, et al. Analysis of a staging assessment system for prediction of surgical interval in recurrent respiratory papillomatosis. Int J Pediatr Otorhinolaryngol 2004;68(12):1493–8.

22. Schraff S, Derkay CS, Burke B, et al. American society of pediatric otolaryngology members' experience with recurrent respiratory papillomatosis and the use of adjuvant therapy. Arch Otolaryngol Head Neck Surg 2004;130:1039–42.

23. Perkins JA, Inglis AF Jr, Richardson MA. Iatrogenic airway stenosis with recurrent respiratory papillomatosis. Arch Otolaryngol Head Neck Surg 1998;124(3): 281–7.
24. Weiss MD, Kashima HK. Tracheal involvement in laryngeal papillomatosis. Laryngoscope 1983;93(1):45–8.
25. Cole RR, Myer CM III, Cotton RT. Tracheotomy in children with recurrent respiratory papillomatosis. Head Neck 1989;11(3):226–30.
26. Shapiro AM, Rimell FL, Shoemaker D, et al. Tracheotomy in children with juvenile-onset recurrent respiratory papillomatosis: the Children's Hospital of Pittsburgh experience. Ann Otol Rhinol Laryngol 1996;105(1):1–5.
27. Chen X, Liu D. The relationship between tracheotomy and intra-tracheal papilloma progression in children. Zhonghua Er Bi Yan Hou Ke Za Zhi 2000;35(5): 384–6.
28. Derkay CS. Recurrent respiratory papillomatosis. Laryngoscope 2001;111(1): 57–69.
29. Zeitels SM, Sataloff RT. Phonomicrosurgical resection of glottal papillomatosis. J Voice 1999;13(1):123–7.
30. Burns JA, Zeitels SM, Akst LM, et al. 532 nm pulsed potassium-titanyl-phosphate laser treatment of laryngeal papillomatosis under general anesthesia. Laryngoscope 2007;117(8):1500–4.
31. Devaiah AK, Shapshay SM, Desai U, et al. Surgical utility of a new carbon dioxide laser fiber: functional and histological study. Laryngoscope 2005;115(8):1463–8.
32. Pasquale K, Wiatrak B, Woolley A, et al. Microdebrider versus CO2 laser removal of recurrent respiratory papillomas: a prospective analysis. Laryngoscope 2003; 113(1):139–43.
33. Mouadeb DA, Belafsky PC. In-office laryngeal surgery with the 585nm pulsed dye laser (PDL). Otolaryngol Head Neck Surg 2007;137(3):477–81.
34. Zeitels SM, Burns JA. Office-based laryngeal laser surgery with the 532-nm pulsed-potassium-titanyl-phosphate laser. Curr Opin Otolaryngol Head Neck Surg 2007;15(6):394–400.
35. Franco RA Jr. In-office laryngeal surgery with the 585-nm pulsed dye laser. Curr Opin Otolaryngol Head Neck Surg 2007;15(6):387–93.
36. McGlennen RC, Adams GL, Lewis CM, et al. Pilot trial of ribavirin for the treatment of laryngeal papillomatosis. Head Neck 1993;15(6):504–12 [discussion: 512–3].
37. Pou AM, Rimell FL, Jordan JA, et al. Adult respiratory papillomatosis: human papillomavirus type and viral coinfections as predictors of prognosis. Ann Otol Rhinol Laryngol 1995;104(10 Pt 1):758–62.
38. Chadha NK, James AL. Antiviral agents for the treatment of recurrent respiratory papillomatosis: a systematic review of the English-language literature. Otolaryngol Head Neck Surg 2007;136(6):863–9.
39. Mandell DL, Arjmand EM, Kay DJ, et al. Intralesional cidofovir for pediatric recurrent respiratory papillomatosis. Arch Otolaryngol Head Neck Surg 2004;130(11): 1319–23.
40. Derkay C. Multi-Disciplinary task force on recurrent respiratory papillomas. Cidofovir for recurrent respiratory papillomatosis (RRP): a re-assessment of risks. Int J Pediatr Otorhinolaryngol 2005;69(11):1465–7.
41. Derkay CS, Faust RA. Recurrent respiratory papillomatosis. In: Cummings CW, Flint PW, Haughey BH, editors. Otolaryngology head and neck surgery. 4th edition. Philadelphia: Mosby, Inc; 2005 [chapter 196]. p. 4370–83.
42. McKenna M, Brodsky L. Extraesophageal acid reflux and recurrent respiratory papilloma in children. Int J Pediatr Otorhinolaryngol 2005;69(5):597–605.

43. Pignatari SS, Liriano RY, Avelino MA, et al. Gastroesophageal reflux in patients with recurrent laryngeal papillomatosis. Rev Bras Otorrinolaringol (Engl Ed) 2007;73(2):210–4.
44. Derkay CS, Smith RJ, McClay J, et al. HspE7 treatment of pediatric recurrent respiratory papillomatosis: final results of an open-label trial. Ann Otol Rhinol Laryngol 2005;114(9):730–7.
45. Kosko JR, Derkay CS. Role of cesarean section in prevention of recurrent respiratory papillomatosis: is there one? Int J Pediatr Otorhinolaryngol 1996;35(1):31–8.
46. Armstrong LR, Derkay CS, Reeves WC. Initial results from the national registry for juvenile-onset recurrent respiratory papillomatosis. RRP Task Force. Arch Otolaryngol Head Neck Surg 1999;125(7):743–8.
47. McNeil C. Who invented the VLP cervical cancer vaccines? J Natl Cancer Inst 2006;98(7):433.
48. Schaffer A, Brotherton J, Booy RJ. Do human papillomavirus vaccines have any role in newborns and the prevention of recurrent respiratory papillomatosis in children? Paediatr Child Health 2007;43(9):579–80.
49. Dasbach EJ, Elbasha EH, Insinga RP. Mathematical models for predicting the epidemiologic and economic impact of vaccination against human papillomavirus infection and disease. Epidemiol Rev 2006;28:88–100.
50. Hill DS, Akhtar S, Corroll A, et al. Quality of life issues in recurrent respiratory papillomatosis. Clin Otolaryngol Allied Sci 2000;25(2):153–60.
51. Lindman JP, Gibbons MD, Morlier R, et al. Voice quality of prepubescent children with quiescent recurrent respiratory papillomatosis. Int J Pediatr Otorhinolaryngol 2004;68(5):529–36.
52. Varni JW, Seid M, Kurtin PS. PedsQL 4.0: reliability and validity of the Pediatric Quality of Life Inventory version 4.0 generic core scales in healthy and patient populations. Med Care 2001;39(8):800–12.
53. Lindman JP, Lewis LS, Accortt N, et al. Use of the pediatric quality of life inventory to assess the health-related quality of life in children with recurrent respiratory papillomatosis. Ann Otol Rhinol Laryngol 2005;114(7):499–503.

Chronic Subjective Dizziness

Michael J. Ruckenstein, MD, MSc, FACS, FRCSC[a],*, Jeffrey P. Staab, MD, MS[a,b]

KEYWORDS

• Dizziness • Vertigo • Anxiety • Migraine

The symptom of dizziness represents a nonspecific complaint that has a broad differential diagnosis. Otolaryngologists naturally focus on the inner ear as the source of the complaint. However, if a patient with dizziness is to be diagnosed accurately and treated effectively, then it is incumbent on the clinician to recognize that dizziness can also be a manifestation of underlying neurological, cardiovascular or psychiatric pathology. In addition, it has long been recognized that psychopathology can produce a sensation of dizziness.[1,2] It is helpful to approach a patient complaining of dizziness in a manner analogous to the approach taken when evaluating a patient presenting with chest pain. Although the initial reflex may be to focus on a cardiac etiology; gastrointestinal, musculoskeletal, and psychologic pathology may also result in chest pain.

It cannot be overemphasized that eliciting a precise description of the dizziness from the patient is the critical factor in delineating the specific diagnosis.[3,4] The specific symptoms described by the patient allow the clinician to categorize the of dizziness (eg, true vertigo, lightheadedness, presyncope, positional imbalance, ataxia); the severity of the dizziness; factors that provoke or ameliorate the dizziness; and any associated symptoms. At times, this description of dizziness is precise and easy to elicit. There are patients, however, who despite the interviewer's best efforts can only describe a vague sensation that defies a precise medical definition. Rather than become frustrated with the patient's inability to articulate a clear description of his or her dizziness, Barber[1] pointed out that such vague symptoms may be evidence, within the first few minutes of the interview, of a psychiatric etiology. Such vague symptoms of chronic heavy headedness, lightheadedness, tightness in the head, and the floor rising and falling are the hallmark of what he and others referred to as "psychogenic dizziness."

[a] Department of Otorhinolaryngology—Head and Neck Surgery, University of Pennsylvania Health System, 3400 Spruce Street, 5 Silverstein, Philadelphia, PA 19104, USA
[b] Department of Psychiatry, Family Medicine and Community Health, University of Pennsylvania Health System, 3535 Market Street, #677, Philadelphia, PA 19104, USA
* Corresponding author.
E-mail address: michael.ruckenstein@uphs.upenn.edu (M.J. Ruckenstein).

Otolaryngol Clin N Am 42 (2009) 71–77
doi:10.1016/j.otc.2008.09.011
0030-6665/08/$ – see front matter © 2009 Elsevier Inc. All rights reserved.

Recognizing that psychiatric factors may have an important role in certain symptoms of dizziness is an important step in counseling patients and avoiding unnecessary medical and surgical procedures. This level of understanding of the disease process, however, has certain limitations. Too often patients are left with the impression that psychogenic dizziness is a diagnosis of exclusion. Simply referring to a process as psychogenic provides no insight as to which of the myriad of potential psychiatric diagnoses are responsible for the symptoms. Furthermore, psychiatric processes may be a cause or consequence of dizziness. They may trigger sensations of dizziness or sustain chronic symptoms following transient medical events. Because successful treatment is predicated on an accurate diagnosis, the need for better diagnostic precision is required.

Approximately 10 years ago the authors set out to better define the entity that was referred to as "psychogenic dizziness." To that end, they endeavored to (1) provide an accurate and reproducible set of diagnostic criteria; (2) delineate the underlying etiologies for the disorder (eg, provide specific psychiatric and medical diagnoses and understand their potential interactions); (3) establish an effective treatment strategy for these patients; and (4) provide a theoretic framework for understanding this disorder that facilitates future research. Their work has resulted in the definition of a clinical entity they refer to as "chronic subjective dizziness" (CSD).

CHRONIC SUBJECTIVE DIZZINESS: SYMPTOMATOLOGY

Patients diagnosed with CSD present with a similar symptom complex:[5,6]

1. Persistent (>3 months) sensation of nonvertiginous dizziness that may include one or more of the following vague descriptors
   a. Lightheadedness
   b. Heavy headedness
   c. A feeling of imbalance that frequently is not apparent to others
   d. A feeling that the "inside of their head" is spinning in the absence of any perception of movement of the visual surround
   e. A feeling that the floor is moving from underneath them
   f. A feeling of disassociation from one's environment
2. Chronic hypersensitivity to one's own motion or the movement of objects in the environment
3. Exacerbation of symptoms in settings with complex visual stimuli, such as grocery stores or shopping malls, or when performing precision visual tasks (eg, working on a computer)

DEMOGRAPHICS

The age range of patients diagnosed with CSD spans from adolescence to late adulthood, but patients are typically between 40 and 50 years of age. Most of the patients (65% to 70%) are women.

CHRONIC SUBJECTIVE DIZZINESS: PATHOGENESIS

Most patients with CSD (93%) have a psychiatric disorder that contributes significantly to their symptoms.[5–8] Based on current classifications in the fourth edition of the *Diagnostic and Statistical Manual of Mental Disorders*, anxiety disorders are by far the most common psychiatric pathology identified, including generalized anxiety disorder, panic or phobic disorders, or minor anxiety (ie, anxiety not otherwise specified in *Diagnostic and Statistical Manual of Mental Disorders-IV*). In a small minority of patients, additional psychiatric pathology was identified including depression, post-traumatic stress disorder, hypochondriasis, and conversion disorder.

The Relationship of Chronic Subjective Dizziness and Other Neuro-Otologic and Neurologic Disorders

The accurate diagnosis of a patient with the complaint of dizziness is dependent on obtaining a precise history and description of the symptoms. It was found that CSD often occurred in patients with a history of a physical neuro-otologic illness (eg, vestibular neuronitis or benign positional vertigo) or neurologic disorder (eg, migraines, postconcussional syndrome).[6] It is particularly important for the clinician to differentiate between symptoms of active neuro-otologic disease (eg, vertigo) and symptoms of CSD (eg, chronic nonvertiginous dizziness). Making this distinction is of immense practical significance. For example, a patient with known Meniere's disease may present complaining of persistent dizziness. Given the patient's known diagnosis, a superficial history of the present complaint may lead the clinician to recommend a vestibuloablative therapy for refractory Meniere's disease. This is more than acceptable if the patient is suffering from vertigo. However, if the patient has actually developed more vague and persistent symptoms consistent with CSD (not an uncommon scenario in patients with Meniere's disease), then vestibuloablative therapy that induces a unilateral vestibular loss could increase his or her anxiety and symptoms. Such a patient might feel worse after treatment, making for an unhappy patient and a frustrated physician. Similarly, in a subset of patients, an episode of vertigo as experienced in benign positional vertigo or vestibular neuronitis may trigger an anxiety response with prolonged symptoms of CSD long after the actual vertigo has resolved.[9] These symptoms persist unless the underlying psychopathology is addressed.

The authors studied the relationship of CSD with other neuro-otologic and neurologic disorders and were able to derive the following classification system.[6,8]

CHRONIC SUBJECTIVE DIZZINESS WITH ANXIETY

A minority of patients with CSD have a primary anxiety disorder. Most have anxiety disorders that are triggered by or coexist with a neuro-otologic illness. The authors found that patients with CSD had one of the following three patterns of presentation.

Otogenic Chronic Subjective Dizziness

These patients had no history of anxiety disorder before developing an acute vestibular insult or other similar pathology (eg, vestibular neuronitis, benign positional vertigo, transient ischemic attack). Their neuro-otologic illness precipitated the onset of anxiety.

Psychogenic Chronic Subjective Dizziness

These patients had no physical disorders including no history of a vestibular disorder. They developed dizziness during the course of their primary anxiety disorder.

Interactive Chronic Subjective Dizziness

These patients had a history of an anxiety disorder or diathesis before the onset of any symptoms of dizziness. They developed CSD and a worsening of their anxiety disorder subsequent to an acute and transient episode of true vertigo or medical condition causing dizziness.

The authors' results indicated that patients were distributed equally between these groups. They reinforce the concept of a bidirectional relationship between dizziness and anxiety: dizziness can cause anxiety and anxiety can cause dizziness. Only one-third of these patients had pure anxiety disorders with no history of physical vestibular disorders. Nevertheless, it must be emphasized that in all these patients, psychiatric processes played the principal role in sustaining both symptoms and functional impairment. Regardless of the subgroup, addressing the psychiatric symptoms in these patients is the key to therapeutic success.

CHRONIC SUBJECTIVE DIZZINESS WITH MIGRAINE

Patients with migraines have an increased incidence of vestibular complaints and anxiety disorders.[10] It was found that close to 20% of patients with CSD had active migraines.[6] This is in keeping with other studies looking at the association between migraines, vestibular complaints, and anxiety. At present, there is general agreement that in patients with these overlapping symptoms, therapeutic interventions must be directed at all the contributing factors, including the migraine headaches, the anxiety disorder, and the vestibular complaints.

CHRONIC SUBJECTIVE DIZZINESS AND OTHER NEUROLOGIC DISORDERS

Patients with postconcussional syndrome represent an enormously challenging group of patients that present with a variety of complaints, including chronic dizziness, depression and irritability, headache, insomnia, and difficulties with memory and concentration. Fifteen percent of the authors' patients with CSD had traumatic brain injury.[6]

Patients with dysautonomias represent a small but significant subgroup of the CSD population.[6,11,12] These patients who have alterations in central neurovascular control can manifest symptoms typical of CSD. At initial evaluation, they can be differentiated from the other subgroups based upon the stimuli that provoke their symptoms. Dysautonomia patients develop CSD with exertion (eg, when engaging in some form of aerobic exercise). Environments that provoke symptoms in CSD with anxiety patients (grocery stores, shopping malls, and so forth) are not as likely to evoke symptoms in patients with dysautonomias.

TREATMENT OF CHRONIC SUBJECTIVE DIZZINESS

Patients with CSD are frustrated and even, at times, desperate. They feel chronically ill and have invariably seen a number of physicians with no benefit. They have tried a variety of medications and other interventions to no avail. They do not receive benefit from traditional interventions for vestibular disease and, as such, some may believe that there is little that can be done to treat their condition. It is in this sense that their treatment may initially be considered palliative. With the interventions outlined below, however, most patients can see a dramatic improvement and even eradication of their symptoms.

Psychoeducation

This is a critical first step in the successful treatment of these patients.[6,13] Many of these patients believe that they have a physical disorder and are reluctant to accept the concept that their symptoms stem from a psychiatric process. As such, a significant period of time must be spent at the initial encounter to educate the patient as to why and how psychologic disease can produce and sustain physical symptoms. This is best performed by a medical professional who is familiar with both the medical and psychiatric aspects of these issues and can spend the required time with the patient.

Putting into place a proper patient education process is critical to the success of the other interventions described next.

Pharmacologic Interventions

The selective serotonin reuptake inhibitors are currently considered to be the first-line therapy for anxiety disorders. The authors and others have evaluated the effects of the selective serotonin reuptake inhibitors on patients with CSD. In a series of open label prospective studies, they found these drugs to be effective in the treatment of CSD.[8,14,15] Roughly 50% of patients studied had a complete remission of symptoms, with approximately 70% showing a significant positive effect. The specific drugs studied and their appropriate doses are listed in **Table 1**. It must be emphasized that when treatment is initiated with selective serotonin reuptake inhibitors, an initial increase in symptoms of anxiety may be observed in patients. This can lead to a premature termination of treatment. It is important to counsel the patient that these effects are typically temporary, and to initiate treatment with low doses that are increased slowly during the first weeks of therapy. Supplementation of the selective serotonin reuptake inhibitors with a benzodiazepine, such as clonazepam, may be beneficial during the initial weeks of treatment. Despite instituting these measures to maximize compliance, roughly 20% of patients in the authors' studies were intolerant of these medications. In patients with migraines and CSD, pharmacotherapy should be directed at addressing both the migraines and the CSD. This may be accomplished with one medication, such as a serotonin norepinephrine reuptake inhibitor (eg, venlafaxine HCl or duloxetine HCl) or possibly a tricyclic antidepressant (eg, nortriptyline). Head trauma patients have multiple central nervous system deficits, as outlined previously. They are best managed in a comprehensive head trauma program that combines pharmacotherapy, neuropsychologic testing and therapy, and physical and occupational therapy.

Behavioral Interventions

Cognitive behavioral therapy is a well-established and effective treatment for patients with anxiety disorders. Its efficacy in treating patients with CSD has not been well established; however, preliminary studies indicate it may be beneficial.[16] Cognitive behavioral therapy is of particular interest in patients with the interactive form of CSD, because they did not respond as well as the other groups of patients to pharmacotherapy alone.

Table 1				
Doses of common selective serotonin reuptake inhibitors				
Drug	Starting Daily Dose (mg)	Target Daily Dose by 4th Week (mg)	Subsequent Daily Increases (at 2—4-Week Intervals) (mg)	Maximum Daily Dose (mg)
Fluoxetine HCl	5–10	20	20	80
Sertraline HCl	12.5–25	50	50	200
Paroxetine HCl	5–10	20	20	60
Citalopram HBr	5–10	20	20	40
Escitalopram oxalate	5	10	10	20
Fluvoxamine maleate	25	150	50	300

Data from Staab JP, Ruckenstein MJ. Chronic dizziness and anxiety: effect of course of illness on treatment outcome. Arch Otolaryngol Head Neck Surg 2005;131:675–9.

Vestibular rehabilitation therapy in which patients are exposed to provocative stimuli in a controlled fashion may have a role for treatment of patients with CSD.[17] Some patients, however, report the exposure to these stimuli to be too uncomfortable and actually report a paradoxical increase in symptoms with vestibular rehabilitation therapy. If vestibular rehabilitation therapy is to be used in this patient group, then it should be administered by a therapist who is sensitive to the severe anxiety response that may be engendered in this patient group when exposed to provocative stimuli.

SUMMARY

Patients with chronic complaints of nonspecific dizziness can present frustrating diagnostic and therapeutic challenges. They seem to have no definite illnesses and seem to be beyond the scope of curative interventions. The authors' work, however, has expanded on previous studies and confirmed that anxiety-related processes cause or maintain symptoms in most cases. Recent research has shown that most patients with these symptoms can be helped by interventions directed at their underlying psychiatric disorders, including current methods of pharmacotherapy and psychotherapy. As a result, patients can be offered definitive, not just palliative, care.

REFERENCES

1. Barber HO. Current ideas on vestibular diagnosis. Otolaryngol Clin North Am 1978;11(2):283–300.
2. Furman JM, Jacob RG. Psychiatric dizziness. Neurology 1997;48(5):1161–6.
3. Baloh RW. Differentiating between peripheral and central causes of vertigo. Otolaryngol Head Neck Surg 1998;119(1):55–9.
4. Ruckenstein MJ. A practical approach to dizziness: questions to bring vertigo and other causes into focus. Postgrad Med 1995;97(3):70–2, 75–8, 81.
5. Ruckenstein MJ, Staab JP. The basic symptom inventory-53 and its use in the management of patients with psychogenic dizziness. Otolaryngol Head Neck Surg 2001;125(5):533–6.
6. Staab JP, Ruckenstein MJ. Expanding the differential diagnosis of chronic dizziness. Arch Otolaryngol Head Neck Surg 2007;133(2):170–6.
7. Staab JP, Ruckenstein MJ. Which comes first? Psychogenic dizziness versus otogenic anxiety. Laryngoscope 2003;113(10):1714–8.
8. Staab JP, Ruckenstein MJ. Chronic dizziness and anxiety: effect of course of illness on treatment outcome. Arch Otolaryngol Head Neck Surg 2005;131(8):675–9.
9. Godemann F, Siefert K, Hantschke-Bruggemann M, et al. What accounts for vertigo one year after euritis vestibularis: anxiety or a dysfunctional vestibular organ? J Psychiatr Res 2005;39(5):529–34.
10. Furman JM, Marcus DA, Balaban CD. Migrainous vertigo: development of a pathogenetic model and structured diagnostic interview. Curr Opin Neurol 2003;16(1):5–13.
11. Staab JP, Ruckenstein MJ, Solomon D, et al. Exertional dizziness and autonomic dysregulation. Laryngoscope 2002;112(8 Pt 1):1346–50.
12. Staab JP, Ruckenstein MJ. Autonomic nervous system function in chronic dizziness. Otol Neurotol 2007;28(6):854–9.
13. Huppert D, Strupp M, Rettinger N, et al. Phobic postural vertigo: a long-term follow-up (5 to 15 years) of 106 patients. J Neurol 2005;252(5):564–9.

14. Staab JP, Ruckenstein MJ, Solomon D, et al. Serotonin reuptake inhibitors for dizziness with psychiatric symptoms. Arch Otolaryngol Head Neck Surg 2002; 128(5):554–60.
15. Staab JP, Ruckenstein MJ, Amsterdam JD. A prospective trial of sertraline for chronic subjective dizziness. Laryngoscope 2004;114(9):1637–41.
16. Holmberg J, Karlberg M, Harlacher U, et al. Treatment of phobic postural vertigo: a controlled study of cognitive-behavioral therapy and self-controlled desensitization. J Neurol 2006;253(4):500–6.
17. Whitney SL, Jacob RG, Sparto PJ, et al. Acrophobia and pathological height vertigo: indications for vestibular physical therapy? Phys Ther 2005;85(5):443–58.

Hearing Loss

Alexa T. Kozak, AuD[a], Kenneth M. Grundfast, MD, FACS[b],*

KEYWORDS

- Hearing loss • Hearing aids • Presbycusis • Autoimmune
- Inner ear disease

Sensorineural hearing loss, depending on rapidity of progression and ultimate severity, can be troublesome, endlessly annoying, and even frightening. Although the otologic surgeon can often operate to improve a conductive hearing impairment or diminish the conductive component of a mixed hearing loss, there really is no surgical procedure that can reverse or lessen the severity of a sensorineural loss. Once a patient is diagnosed with progressive sensorineural hearing loss, some therapeutic interventions can be used but there is little certainty that any single intervention will reliably improve or preserve hearing. Even though administering steroids and antimetabolites may be helpful for some patients diagnosed with autoimmune inner ear disease, in most cases when the otolaryngologist is managing a patient with sensorineural hearing loss, therapy is directed more toward helping the patient cope with the loss of hearing rather than offering various medical or surgical interventions that are expected to induce the physiologic changes necessary to improve their hearing acuity. Accordingly, for the patient with sensorineural hearing loss, the care plan is usually more directed toward palliation than toward cure.

This article views hearing loss not only as a physiologic deficit measurable numerically in decibels, but as the loss of an important aspect of overall communication skill that can have far reaching emotional and psychologic effects on the patient, the family, and those who surround patients in their daily lives. Although there is little otolaryngologists and audiologists can do reliably to restore lost sensorineural components of hearing, and although collectively they are unable to abate the progression of sensorineural hearing loss, typically described as presbycusis, this article does offer strategies for managing the patient who is losing or who has lost hearing.

HEARING LOSS: AN OVERVIEW

The term "sensorineural" is used here to describe the hearing loss that is believed to be the result of a physiologic malfunction in the inner ear or acoustic nerve. The

[a] Division of Audiology, Boston University School of Medicine and the Boston Medical Center, Boston, MA, USA
[b] Department Otolaryngology-Head and Neck Surgery, Boston University School of Medicine and the Boston Medical Center, FGH Building, Suite 4500, 820 Harrison Avenue, Boston, MA 02118, USA
* Corresponding author.
E-mail address: kenneth.grundfast@bmc.org (K.M. Grundfast).

Otolaryngol Clin N Am 42 (2009) 79–85
doi:10.1016/j.otc.2008.09.008
0030-6665/08/$ – see front matter © 2009 Published by Elsevier Inc.
oto.theclinics.com

"sensory" component of the hearing loss conceptually correlates with malfunction in the organ of Corti, likely within the hair cells, and becomes manifest when elevated puretone thresholds are seen on an audiogram. The neural component conceptually correlates with malfunction within or proximate to the acoustic nerve and is recognizable when a patient has poor word discrimination when tested by an audiologist. For example, if a patient with moderate sensorineural hearing loss based on puretone scores has excellent word discrimination scores, this suggests that the locus of the problem is more within the inner ear than in the acoustic nerve or in the brain. For a patient who has a mild to moderate sensorineural hearing loss along with poor word discrimination, however, this suggests that the patient might have problems both within the inner ear and also perhaps within the acoustic nerve, and possibly the patient may also be experiencing difficulty with brain function. In general, people with hearing impairment mostly confined to the inner ear do well with amplification and hearing aids, whereas those who have impaired function of the acoustic nerve and impaired brain function typically have more difficulty using hearing aids.

Sensorineural hearing loss can vary with respect to onset and severity, and can affect one or both ears. The onset of the hearing loss is typically defined as prelingual if it manifests before speech-language acquisition and defined as postlingual if is known to have occurred after speech development. It should be noted that all congenital hearing loss is prelingual but not all prelingual hearing loss is congenital. Hearing loss that develops after birth is generally referred to as "acquired" hearing loss. Congenital hearing loss usually is the result of a prenatal infection, such as rubella, toxoplasmosis, cytomegalovirus, or herpes, or the hearing loss can be inherited as a result of a gene mutation. Acquired hearing loss in children might be caused by meningitis or some injury to the inner ear including the effect of receiving ototoxic medication. Acquired hearing loss in adults is usually attributed to noise exposure, trauma, ototoxic drugs, presbycusis, or Meniere's disease. Some adults develop sudden hearing loss with no apparent cause, and this is described as sudden idiopathic sensorineural hearing loss. Hearing loss usually is bilateral and symmetrical; however, in the case of Meniere's disease and sudden sensorineural hearing loss, the disease process may produce a unilateral hearing loss. Often in the case of unilateral hearing loss, the patient may experience the feeling of being off balance and lack the ability correctly to localize sound. Frequently, patients who have an acquired unilateral hearing loss are faced with the unknown in regards to the other ear. Many times, their first question is if they will develop a hearing loss in the other ear. Counseling and palliative care are essential in caring for and treating these patients.

Sensorineural hearing loss can develop then progress over time, and is seen commonly in genetic- and syndrome-associated hearing loss, presbycusis, autoimmune inner ear disease, and Meniere's disease. Approximately 70% of genetic hearing loss is nonsyndromic,[1,2] whereas the remaining 30% is considered to be syndromic because it is associated with findings that can be detected on physical examination. Over 400 genetic syndromes that include hearing loss have been described.[3] Syndromic hearing loss constitutes approximately 30% of prelingual deafness; however, its overall contribution to all hearing loss is much smaller, reflecting the occurrence and diagnosis of postlingual and often progressive hearing loss (Stickler's syndrome, Usher syndrome, Alport's syndrome). Presbycusis is hearing loss related to aging and is typically associated with high-frequency hearing loss and compromised speech intelligibility. Patients report that they can hear what people are saying but they are having a difficult time understanding what is being said. Many patients with presbycusis benefit from amplification and successfully use hearing aids. The hearing loss associated with autoimmune inner ear disease and Meniere's disease, however, tends to fluctuate and worsen over time. Autoimmune inner ear disease is difficult to diagnose because there really is no single reliable laboratory test to confirm the diagnosis. In general, a hearing loss that occurs relatively rapidly in one or both ears especially in young or middle aged adults potentially could be autoimmune inner ear disease. If the hearing improves with steroid medication given orally, then this further suggests an autoimmune etiology. When patients have repeatedly had hearing improvement while on steroids and then decrement in hearing after cessation of the steroid medication, then low-dose methotrexate therapy can be considered for long-term management instead of leaving the patient on the steroid.[4] Unfortunately, despite medical treatment, patients with autoimmune inner ear disease can have progressive hearing loss leading to deafness. Because there is no treatment that can reliably restore hearing or maintain improved hearing long-term, the management of autoimmune inner ear disease is palliative, not curative. Patients with autoimmune inner ear disease usually have lived most of their lives with normal hearing and they become quite upset when they realize that they have a condition that can result in severe hearing impairment perhaps jeopardizing their employment and creating, for them, major communication problems.

EFFECTS OF HEARING LOSS

Hearing loss affects not only the patient, but also loved ones and anyone whom the patient must communicate with in daily life. In general, younger patients with difficulty hearing often experience frustration, depression, and anxiety related to the loss of hearing. More elderly patients with presbycusis tend to view the hearing loss as part of the process of aging, and they seem to accept the hearing loss as just something that happens and can be accepted. Interestingly, not all patients who have hearing impairment are eager to obtain a hearing aid. Some patients say that amplification does not work because one of their friends had a bad experience with a hearing aid, or say that they cannot afford to purchase a hearing aid because most insurance companies do not reimburse for the costs of hearing aids. When a loved one or family member has hearing impairment severe enough to affect conversation but the patient is reluctant to obtain a hearing aid, then this can cause frustration within the family.

Much like the well known stages of accepting that an illness is terminal and incurable, patients diagnosed with presbysusis or progressive hearing loss can go through stages of acceptance of their disability analogous to the Kübler-Ross stages of death and dying (**Box 1**).

The stages shown in the box below describe the emotions of individuals dealing with grief and loss. They were originally applied to those who experienced catastrophic personal loss; however, others have applied them to considerable personal changes. Kübler-Ross[5] stated that the stages do not necessarily occur in this order, nor are they experienced by all persons; however, individuals tend to experience at least two of the stages.

When a child is born deaf, then the parents go through an adjustment period, first perhaps being in denial and then finally accepting that their child will be unable to hear normally and perhaps become optimistic that a cochlear implant will help their child to live a near normal life. During the stage of denial, parents confronted with results of a follow-up newborn hearing test indicating significant hearing impairment may question the accuracy of the test because they believe their child is responding to his or her name or the child can hear sounds in the home. Ultimately, parents are able to accept the reality that they have a hearing impaired child. The roles of the physician and audiologist in working with the parents of a hearing impaired child are to be

---

Box 1
Stages of acceptance of progressive hearing loss

Denial: the initial stage. "This can't be happening." "I can hear fine but my spouse and other folks just aren't speaking as clearly as they used to talk"

Anger: "Why me/my child/my loved one? This is not fair!" (referring to oneself, God, or anyone perceived as "responsible") "Why don't people just speak up and look at me when they are speaking?,"People are so impatient, if I ask someone to repeat what is being said or to raise the volume of their voice just a little, they act indignant—what's that all about?"

Bargaining: "Just let me lose a little bit of my hearing, not all of it," or "Just let my child have hearing until they learn speech/language." I would like to get by without a hearing aid just a little bit longer. I know that a hearing aid might be helpful, but can I wait about a year or so to see what happens and then reconsider using a hearing aid? I'm just not ready for a hearing aid now"

Depression: "I am never going to have a normal life again," or "my child is never going to be normal or be successful." I will never again be able to hear the music I used to love— this is terrible.

Acceptance: "I will manage and do what I can to regain some normalcy." Or "I will do anything so that my child will succeed in academics and life."

---

supportive, to listen to the concerns of the parents, and to assist the parents in deciding what choices to make among the many alternatives for management of the child's hearing impairment. Parents need to be guided through the process of pursuing and obtaining the appropriate accommodations, such as hearing and speech evaluations and individualized education plans. As parents cope with the stress of realizing and accepting that they have a hearing impaired child, making the difficult choices needed how best to be of help to their child, puts considerable stress on the entire family.[6] Although hearing impairment can be helped but not cured, the well-being of the affected child and the involved family depends greatly on a team of involved professionals including an otolaryngologist or otologist, an audiologist, and a speech-language pathologist who are able to be supportive, listen to the concerns being expressed, and provide guidance.

In contrast to the situation surrounding the birth of a hearing impaired child, when a young patient develops hearing loss that was not present at birth there is a tendency for the affected patient to experience grief related to the loss of hearing. That is, the child or young adult who is experiencing loss of hearing after having previously had normal hearing must cope with a major change in self-image and daunting challenges in ability to perform daily activities. The management of a child or young adult with progressive sensorineural hearing loss can be one of the most frustrating aspects of practicing otolaryngology because explaining the cause of such hearing loss is difficult and there is so little that can be done medically or surgically to restore hearing or even to avert further hearing loss. Consequently, otolaryngologists and audiologists managing the patient need to be supportive and optimistic about the ultimate outcome for the patient without providing misleading information that can give the patients and parents false hope. In past decades, parents of children and young adults who were experiencing progressive sensorineural hearing loss were told that the hearing loss might be caused by a perilymph fistula and exploration of the middle ear, with repair of the fistula if found, could restore hearing or prevent further loss of hearing. During that bygone era in otology, too many parents were given false hopes about the benefits of a simple surgical procedure and too many youngsters had surgical procedures that probably were not needed or even helpful. Fortunately, that era in the management of progressive sensorineural hearing loss has ended and it is now known that the palliative care for patients with progressive hearing loss mostly involves emotional support, genetic testing, discussions about amplification with hearing aids, and cochlear implants, not talk of quick operations with little proved benefit. Information helpful in having rational and reasonable discussions with families about the kinds of hearing loss that cannot be corrected with middle ear surgery is discussed next.

OPTIONS

It is important to educate the patient and their families on the nature and treatment of progressive sensorineural hearing loss. Clear explanations should be provided of the potential risks regarding all medical treatment options, such as orally administered steroid or transtympanic injection of steroid.

Hearing Aids

One of the most common and noninvasive ways of managing a patient with hearing loss is fitting them with hearing aids. In recent years, rapid advancements in technology have made hearing aids a more viable option for patients. Digital technology provides the patient options and enables them to give feedback regarding the sound quality. Patient feedback allows the audiologist the ability to make appropriate changes, making the hearing loss more manageable and their lives more enjoyable. Even with the option to change and adjust the hearing aids, the success of the hearing aid is dependant on several factors. One factor is affordability of the hearing aids. Medicare and most private insurances do not provide financial coverage or subsequent monies to help defer the cost of hearing aids. Medicaid typically covers the cost of the device; however, the benefit policies vary by state. A second factor is the patient's motivation and willingness to wear the hearing aid. If a patient believes that they do not have a hearing loss or they do not need a hearing aid, their acceptance of the hearing aid is compromised. A third factor is the patient's word discrimination abilities. If a patient has poor word discrimination, a hearing aid is only going to amplify sounds and provide minimal benefit in regards to speech intelligibility. It is here that the patient needs to be counseled thoroughly on the limitations of hearing aids. Often patients tend to associate vision and hearing together (glasses and hearing aids); an analogy of macular degeneration and glasses can be given to patients to illustrate the limits of hearing aids. More specifically, if the person who has macular degeneration wears glasses, that person can still see objects, but the objects are not seen clearly.

Cochlear Implants

Cochlear implantation may be an option when hearing aids no longer provide ample benefit for the patient because of the severity of loss. Because cochlear implantation is becoming a more accepted surgery, patients are more likely to view the surgery as routine and may not realize the full breadth of what is involved. It is essential that the scope of the surgery and the required postoperative and follow-up visits for mapping be explained to the patient and the family.

As with hearing aids, cochlear implant technology has become increasingly sophisticated; nonetheless, there continues to be limitations. Frequently, patients who were post-lingually deafened state that the auditory signal sounds artificial and robotic. There have been many studies that have examined the factors affecting auditory performance and the wide variability in the speech recognition performance of cochlear implant patients.[7–9] Duration of deafness, age of onset of deafness, age at implantation, and other factors, such as number of surviving spiral ganglion cells, electrode placement and depth, and signal processing strategy, effect the success of the patient. More specifically, individuals who have been deaf for a shorter period of time and have experienced less auditory deprivation tend to attain better speech performance scores then those who have been deaf for a longer time. It has also been established that patients who are postlingually deaf perform better than those who are prelingually deaf. Depending on the placement of the electrode and the patient's anatomy, some electrodes may need to be disabled because of stimulation of the facial nerve, compromising the full potential of the implant. Nonauditory-related factors including, aural rehabilitation, the patient's dedication to the program, and familial support all play a role.

Assistive Listening Devices

Assistive listening technologies can be used in conjunction with hearing aids and cochlear implants. Assistive listening devices include but are not limited to FM systems; amplified telephones; alerting signals (doorbells, vibrating alarm clocks, smoke detectors); and telecommunication device for the deaf (TTY-TDD). FM systems range from large area coverage, such as loop induction and infrared systems, to smaller range area coverage, such as personal FM systems. FM systems are recommended for school-aged children because they provide the child with a better signal-to-noise ratio. This allows the child to focus their attention on the information coming directly from the teacher. FM systems are also recommended for individuals who struggle to understand speech in noise. Although many hearing aids come with a telecoil, which aids in communication on the telephone, an amplified phone can provide the extra boost in volume that the patient is looking for. Alerting signals, such as a flashing light in place of an audible doorbell or smoke alarm, can ensure the patient's safety in the home. TTY-TDD are still used; however, computer programs, such as e-mail, instant messenger, and text messaging, are replacing the use of the TTY-TDD because of the cost and cumbersome nature of the device.

COUNSELING

Counseling both the patient and the family on hearing loss and providing them with communication techniques can help alleviate some of their fears. There are some simple, everyday suggestions that can facilitate communication: making sure that the speaker has the attention of the listener; facing the hearing impaired individual while speaking so that they are maximizing auditory and visual cues; or strategic seating while in a restaurant, for example sitting away from the kitchen or sitting with one's back to the wall. It is also important to educate the patient on noise precautions and hearing protection. Audiologists can better assist and manage in the habilitation or rehabilitation of the person who is hearing impaired. In the case of children, audiologists recognize the importance of a comprehensive evaluation to make certain they are receiving the appropriate services, such as amplification, speech therapy, and educational services. With adults, they can discuss amplification and speech reading classes.

In the end, after providing all of the treatment options, one of the most important components in dealing with patients or families who experience hearing loss is to offer the option of counseling. During the grieving process individuals can feel alone, and ensuring that they have someone to talk to about their feelings allows them to be more open and accepting of their situation. Additionally, providing information about support groups helps the individual feel less isolated.

SUMMARY

Progressive hearing loss affects not only the patient, but directly impacts the family of the patient. Although conductive hearing impairment caused by middle ear effusion associated with otitis media, stapes fixation from otosclerosis, or ossicular discontinuity from trauma or sequela of otitis media can be corrected and effectively cured with surgery, there really is not a medical or surgical way to reliably reverse or prevent progression of sensorineural hearing loss once it has become manifest. Consequently, much of the management of a child or an adult with sensorineural hearing loss involves providing care that does not bring about actual hearing improvement, but instead helps the patient and family to live the best lives possible despite the loss of hearing. Once the diagnosis of sensorineural hearing impairment is made, the thrust of management is toward palliation and coping rather than toward fixing the malfunction within the ear or other parts of the auditory system.

RELATED READINGS

Schow RL, Nerbonne MA. Introduction to audiologic rehabilitation: 3rd edition. Simon and Schuster. 1996.
Smith RJH, van Camp G. Deafness and hereditary hearing loss overview. Available at: http://www.geneclinics.org/profiles/deafness-overview/details.html. Accessed September 30, 2007.

REFERENCES

1. Cremers CW, Marres HA, van Rijn PM. Nonsyndromal profound genetic deafness in childhood. Ann N Y Acad Sci 1991;630:191–6.
2. van Camp G, Willems PJ, Smith RJ. Nonsyndromic hearing impairment: unparalleled heterogeneity. Am J Hum Genet 1997;60:758–64.
3. Gorlin RJ, Toriello HV, Cohen MM, editors. Hereditary hearing loss and its syndromes. New York: Oxford University Press; 1995.
4. Salley LH Jr, Grimm M, Sismanis A, et al. Methotrexate in the management of immune mediated cochleovestibular disorders: clinical experience with 53 patients. J Rheumatol 2001;28:1037–40.
5. Kübler-Ross E. On death and dying. New York: Simon & Schuster; 1997.
6. Aronson J. Sound and fury. Aronson film Associates, Inc. and Public Policy Productions, Inc. in association with Thirteen/WNET New York, 2001.
7. Gantz B, Woodworth G, Abbas P, et al. Multivariate predictors of audiological success with multichannel cochlear implants. Ann Otol Rhinol Laryngol 1993;102: 909–16.
8. Summerfield A, Marshall D. Preoperative predictors of outcomes from cochlear implantation in adults: performance and quality of life. Ann Otol Rhinol Laryngol 1995;Supplement 166:105–8.
9. Blamey P, Arndt P, Bergeron F, et al. Factors affecting auditory performance of postlinguistically deaf adults using cochlear implants. Audiol and NeuroOtol 1996;1:293–306.

Disorders of Swallowing: Palliative Care

Susan E. Langmore, PhD*, Gregory Grillone, MD, FACS,
Alphi Elackattu, MD, Michael Walsh, MA

KEYWORDS

- Dysphagia • Deglutition disorders • Behavioral treatment
- Surgical treatment • Palliative care

Dysphagia, or difficulty swallowing, occurs commonly, especially in elderly and debilitated patients. The exact prevalence of dysphagia is unknown, but some reports suggest that the prevalence could be as high as 22% in persons aged more than 50 years.[1] Approximately 10 million people are evaluated annually in the United States for swallowing difficulties.[2] Several studies conclude that between 300,000 and 600,000 individuals in the United States are affected by neurogenic causes of dysphagia each year.[3] Within the hospital setting, many persons experience dysphagia due to general weakness, debilitation, severe pulmonary disease, intubation, or a reduced level of alertness. These numbers clearly indicate a significant burden for treatment teams and patients alike.

This article defines palliative care for swallowing disorders as treatment for severe and chronic dysphagia or intractable aspiration when the recovery of normal swallowing is not anticipated and attempts to restore normal swallowing have been unsuccessful. Palliative treatment for dysphagia is not only for the dying patient because patients with difficulty swallowing can live for a long time. The focus herein is on a variety of common causes for stable or progressive swallowing dysfunction. Palliative care for dysphagia is aimed at maximizing swallowing function, maintaining pulmonary health, and supporting healthy nutrition despite the impaired ability to swallow. When despite all attempts at intervention a patient becomes totally unable to swallow, the goal of therapy changes toward finding ways to provide adequate nutrition for the patient.

Department of Otolaryngology, Boston University Medical Center, FGH Building, 4th floor, Harrison Street, Boston, MA 02118, USA
* Corresponding author.
E-mail address: langmore@bu.edu (S.E. Langmore).

Otolaryngol Clin N Am 42 (2009) 87–105
doi:10.1016/j.otc.2008.09.005
0030-6665/08/$ – see front matter © 2009 Elsevier Inc. All rights reserved.

oto.theclinics.com

NORMAL SWALLOWING MECHANISM

The act of swallowing can be divided into oral, pharyngeal, and esophageal phases. The initial oral phase is mainly voluntary and includes putting food or liquid in the mouth, preparing it, and then transporting it to the pharynx. In addition to motor ability, food consistency, taste, hunger, and motivation affect the efficiency of the oral phase. The pharyngeal phase consists of several coordinated actions which transport the food from the oropharynx to the esophagus. This phase can occur involuntarily but may also be modified volitionally via cortical and subcortical input. The esophageal phase is strictly involuntary and partly under autonomic control. This article concentrates solely on oral and pharyngeal, or oropharyngeal, dysphagia.

STANDARD DYSPHAGIA THERAPY

Before discussing palliative care for dysphagia, the standard approach to helping all patients who are experiencing difficulty swallowing is reviewed. In most cases of oropharyngeal dysphagia, there is an underlying medical or functional cause for the problem which must be determined before appropriate treatment can be pursued. If the underlying medical condition is permanent or progressive, a chronic type of dysphagia may be present. Surgery and medications may lessen the swallowing problem, but behavioral and dietary treatments are often the most effective intervention techniques. Speech-language pathologists are the specialists who are trained to evaluate and treat dysphagia with behavioral techniques.

Compensatory

Interventions that are intended to compensate for the problem are compensatory in nature. Examples of compensatory techniques are diet modifications (eg, eliminate hard, chewy food or thin liquids), postural changes (eg, tuck in the chin when swallowing),[4] alterations in swallowing behavior (eg, swallowing three times to clear the residue before taking the next bite), or external manipulations (eg, taking liquids from a spoon).[5] Most of these techniques are aimed at reducing the bolus size or redirecting the bolus path and protecting the airway to prevent aspiration and improve bolus clearance; however, they are all "immediate fixes" that need to be employed consistently to work. Another type of compensatory treatment is the use of dental appliances in the mouth. These devices are useful to occlude nasopharyngeal defects and assist the tongue with bolus propulsion. Any of these compensatory interventions may be useful in a patient who has chronic severe dysphagia.

Rehabilitative

Rehabilitative interventions are meant to improve the underlying ability of the person to swallow faster, stronger, or in a timelier manner.[6-8] The long-term goal is to improve the swallow without the need for any intervention. Prime examples of these interventions are exercises for the tongue, larynx, or pharynx.[9-11] Research has proven the benefit of several of these exercises; however, it takes a compliant cooperative patient with the endurance to undertake the exercises for them to be practical. These interventions also require that the underlying medical condition will not make exercise counterproductive (eg, will lead to fatigue without improvement in strength).

Compensatory/Rehabilitative

Some interventions have immediate positive effects on swallowing efficiency or safety but may also change the long-term ability of the person to swallow better. These interventions are compensatory when first introduced but may be rehabilitative in the long run. Examples are the use of increased sensory stimulation (ice, sour taste, thermal stimulation, electrical stimulation) or the use of swallow maneuvers that require effort on the part of the patient (Mendelsohn maneuver, effortful swallow, or suprasuperglottic swallow).[12–14] These interventions have been shown to have immediate positive effects on the swallow, but their permanent effect has yet to be tested.[15]

CHRONIC DYSPHAGIA AFTER HEAD AND NECK CANCER

A patient with cancer of the head and neck who undergoes extirpative surgery is likely to have impairment of function of nerves and muscles that control swallowing. After the immediate effects of the chemotherapy, radiotherapy, and surgery subside, a chronic dysphagia may become apparent. Patients may be free of cancer, but their quality of life can be significantly reduced. Before these long-term issues are addressed, a brief review of the most common problems is in order.

Oral Cancer

Severe swallowing disorders of the oral tongue may persist following surgical resection of the mobile tongue if grafts or free flaps are adynamic, the anterior tongue is tethered to the floor of the mouth, or the tongue is immobile secondary to hypoglossal nerve resection. Obviously, the person will not be able to masticate adequately or move the bolus out of the mouth. Pauloski and colleagues[16] found that aspiration was not a common occurrence after surgery of the oral tongue unless removal extended deep into the floor of the mouth including the geniohyoid and mylohyoid muscles, affecting the pharyngeal stage of swallowing.[17]

Oropharyngeal Cancer

Resection of tumors of the tonsil and base of tongue affect the pharyngeal phase of swallowing and increase the risk of aspiration. Logemann and colleagues[18,19] found that patients with resection of the tongue base had difficulty initiating the swallow and slowed pharyngeal transit time. Zuydam and colleagues[20] reported that patients with more than 25% of the tongue base resected experienced great swallowing difficulty, with postoperative aspiration a particular concern.

Laryngeal Cancer

Surgical resection of stage III and IV cancers of the larynx often adversely affects swallowing and airway protection. Tumors of the epiglottis, aryepiglottic folds, and false vocal folds may require a supraglottic laryngectomy. Because these structures are involved in the protection of the airway, their removal increases the risk of aspiration. When the resection needs to be extended into the tongue base or to the arytenoids, aspiration during the swallow is the likely consequence.[15] Supracricoid laryngectomy predisposes patients to swallowing disorders and aspiration.[21]

Radio Therapy

Radiotherapy to the oral, pharyngeal, and laryngeal cavities often causes early difficulty in swallowing due to mucositis, odynophagia, trismus, loss of taste, and alteration in saliva.[15] Although these effects generally subside within a few months after radiotherapy, the late effects of therapy may persist for months or years, leaving a chronic severe dysphagia that may grow worse over time. The toxicity will be worsened with higher doses of radiotherapy or with the addition of chemotherapy.[22–24] Postradiation edema and radiation-induced fibrosis of the oropharyngeal musculature lead to noncompliance of tissue and immobility of underlying muscles. These changes result in significant difficulty moving the bolus through the pharynx and closing off of the airway, leaving residue within the pharynx and increasing aspiration.[25–29] Logemann and colleagues[30] reported similar findings in patients treated with various chemoradiation protocols.

Patients with dysphagia following head and neck cancer may be able to execute swallowing maneuvers that keep the bolus out of the airway (eg, the suprasupraglottic swallow), and they may be able to maintain an oral diet if they can clear residue of food with liquids without aspirating. Nevertheless, these maneuvers may be impossible for older, more severe, or more fragile patients. When weight loss and recurrent pneumonias become evident, it may be time to consider alternate treatments.

CHRONIC DYSPHAGIA IN PROGRESSIVE NEUROLOGIC DISEASE
Amyotrophic Lateral Sclerosis

Amyotrophic lateral sclerosis (ALS) is a progressive motor neuron disease of undetermined etiology. Presentation normally occurs during the fifth to eighth decade. Male patients outnumber females 2 to 1. The prevalence is estimated at 2 to 7 cases per 100,000 persons. The disease process involves degeneration of upper (UMN) and lower (LMN) motor neurons within the cortex, brainstem, and spinal cord. Presentation varies depending on the initial site of involvement. Patients with spinal onset (approximately 70%) present with limb symptoms such as muscle atrophy, weakness, spasticity, or stumbling. Approximately 30% of patients present with bulbar onset which initially affects speech, swallowing, and voice.[31] If UMN symptoms predominate, slowed slurred speech is the initial symptom, whereas if LMN involvement is dominant, swallowing difficulties may emerge before speech is noticeably worse. As the disease progresses, both UMN and LMN damage are present.

In general, the incidence of dysphagia in this population tends to be high. Virtually all patients experience swallowing problems at some point in the disease if they live long enough. There is evidence that patients may benefit from swallowing therapy early on in the course of the disease.[32] As the dysphagia becomes severe, aspiration pneumonia becomes a greater threat; however, the most frequent cause of death is ventilatory failure due to palsy of the respiratory muscles; 50% of patients with bulbar onset die within 3 years of diagnosis.[33]

Standard swallowing assessments for ALS patients rely on a clinical, videofluoroscopic, or laryngoscopic procedure to assess the severity of the problem. In the authors' experience, corroborated by Leder,[34] fiberoptic endoscopic evaluation of swallowing is a patient-friendly assessment procedure that can be done conveniently in the clinic and provides immediate visual biofeedback for the patient and family. Standard therapy for dysphagia in ALS emphasizes compensatory interventions such as postural changes and diet modifications. Swallowing exercises are contraindicated due to excess fatigue and the lack of evidence for any benefit. Compensatory techniques are the mainstay until the patient cannot take anything by mouth without choking and aspirating.

Both assessment and therapy need to take the cognitive status of the ALS patient into consideration, because approximately one third of patients and nearly one half of bulbar onset patients have some degree of frontotemporal lobar dementia (FTLD).[35] These patients may not recognize or self-report their swallowing problems, nor will they monitor their ability to swallow safely. It is important to work closely with the caretakers of ALS patients with dementia to guide them in helping the patient compensate for the specific deficits.

Parkinson's Disease

Parkinson's disease is an idiopathic, progressive, neuromuscular disorder that affects about 2 million people in America.[36] The cardinal symptoms of tremor, rigidity, and bradykinesia are due to alterations in neural circuits within the basal ganglia that regulate movement. These changes are correlated with loss of pigmented dopaminergic cells in the pars compacta region of the substantia nigra. The average life expectancy of a patient who has Parkinson's disease is generally lower than for people who do not have the disease, but the progression of symptoms may take 20 years or more. The reported incidence of swallowing dysfunction in Parkinson's disease ranges from 30% to 52%, with symptoms correlating with disease severity and duration.[37]

The cardinal symptoms of akinesia, bradykinesia, and rigidity are responsible for the dysphagia in Parkinson's disease. Some of the salient symptoms are inefficient vertical chewing movements, an open mouth posture with anterior leakage of the bolus, delayed and uncoordinated lingual posterior thrust of the bolus into the pharynx, and delayed triggering of the swallow reflex. Pharyngeal clearance and laryngeal valving may appear weak, and bolus clearance is reduced. Potulska and colleagues[38] quantified several of these problems in a study comparing Parkinson's disease patients with controls. Interestingly, they reported that dysphagia was observed in all 18 patients studied, even though only 13 complained about it. Subclinical dysphagia may be one of the early symptoms of Parkinson's disease.

Behavioral management of the dysphagia can prove useful in the early stages of Parkinson's disease. In addition to compensatory strategies, exercise is recommended and may even retard progression of the swallowing disorder;[39] however, this has not been proven in a controlled study. Later in the course of the disease, exercise is no longer effective, and compensatory diet and postural changes may be of some benefit. In some patients, dysphagia becomes so severe that feeding tubes are the only option to weight loss and aspiration-related complications. Because the disease progresses slowly, many patients and families opt to continue to eat orally until the end. With careful feeding, they may succeed in this strategy. Others opt for supplemental tube feeding but retaining some oral feeding for pleasure. Quality of life is the preeminent concern at this stage.

Most studies enforce the idea that levodopa and deep brain stimulation are usually beneficial for treating limb motor signs associated with this disease; however, there is no equivalent improvement in dysarthria and dysphagia with these same interventions.[40] One exception to this finding is the study by Bushman and colleagues[41] who demonstrated improved swallowing with the use of levodopa in 7 of 20 patients.

The authors' clinical experience with Parkinson's disease patients suggests that they do not generally seek out treatment for dysphagia until it is severe. Voice problems are usually more troublesome for the patient. If the voice therapy can include some general tongue, laryngeal, and pharyngeal strengthening exercises, this may benefit swallowing, but this impression needs to be investigated carefully in a controlled study.

The Dementias

Dementia is a pathologic disorder defined by an acquired and progressive deficit in one or more major cognitive functions. The most common of these is Alzheimer's disease, which according to the Centers for Disease Control[42] affects about 4 million Americans, with 370,000 new cases a year. Other types include vascular, Lewy body, and FTLD. The dysphagia seen across these disorders is similar in many respects; therefore, it is addressed herein with regard to the most common etiology of Alzheimer's disease.

Aspiration pneumonia has been reported to be the most common cause of mortality in various forms of dementia.[43,44] In addition to dysphagia, other conditions that predispose to aspiration pneumonia include a reduced level of consciousness, a bed-bound state, dependency for activities of daily living, advanced age, periodontal disease, and the effects of various tubes in the respiratory and gastrointestinal tracts leaving patients vulnerable to indigenous and nosocomial flora. The presence of dysphagia in late-stage dementia was well described by Feinberg and colleagues[45] who evaluated oral and pharyngeal function in 131 institutionalized elderly patients with advanced dementia with videofluoroscopic swallow studies. In fact, objective findings were normal in only nine (7%) patients. Priefer and colleagues[46] discovered that dysphagia may manifest early on in the disease process in patients with dementia. Similarly, patients with early FTLD may manifest swallowing deficits that generally go unrecognized,[47] which may be due to the more obvious aberrant eating behaviors that these patients often display, such as rapid compulsive eating. As the dementia progresses, dysphagia is more apparent, especially when motor problems are a part of the diagnosis, such as in progressive supranuclear palsy.

As is true for other disorders, management of dysphagia in dementia is complicated. Little evidence suggests that aspiration can be prevented by standard management techniques, and the beneficial role of enteral feeding in patients with advanced dementia has not been shown. There is much debate regarding the benefits and risks of long-term enteral feeding in these patients. Patients on enteral nutrition are still at increased risk of pneumonia from aspiration of saliva or gastroesophageal reflux.

Cerebrovascular Disease

Cerebrovascular accidents are devastating occurrences that can have life-altering consequences. There were projected to be 750,000 strokes in 2007,[48] and approximately 4.6 million Americans are currently living post stroke.[49] The morbidity and mortality of cerebrovascular accidents are significant, with a 1-month fatality rate of about 23%. For patients with dysphagia, the mortality rate is even higher, that is, 37% to 42%. After acute stroke, 27% to 50% of patients have dysphagia, including up to 50% of the stroke neurorehabilitation population.[50–52] Swallowing abnormalities in stroke are variable and may include oral food retention, delayed oral transfer, delayed elicitation of a pharyngeal swallow, decreased hyolaryngeal elevation, and aspiration.[53]

Dysphagia manifestations, severity, and prognosis are greatly affected by the locus of neurologic damage. Several investigators have disputed the notion that only bilateral strokes can lead to dysphagia, although the nature of the problem varies with the site of lesion. In general, anterior and subcortical strokes result in a high rate of dysphagia,[54–56] whereas brainstem stroke typically causes the most severe dysphagia, especially if the medulla is affected.[57,58] Patients with the right hemisphere affected may manifest behavioral deficits that reduce their ability to use compensatory strategies taught to them.[53]

Recovery of dysphagia from a cerebrovascular accident varies depending on the area affected. Meng and coworkers found that although 81% of the patients had dysphagia at the time of initial clinical swallowing evaluation, 88% of the patients resumed full oral intake 4 months after the onset of stroke.[59] Generally, if swallowing function is going to recover it will do so within 6 or 7 weeks after a stroke.[53] Brainstem stroke, bilateral hemispheric involvement, or multiple cortical strokes may take longer to recover and may result in a permanent dysphagia. These patients need palliative care when standard treatment fails. Because they have a stable dysphagia and may live many years after the stroke, care is particularly frustrating. Finding food or liquid that they can take orally enhances quality of life immensely. Exercise may help at later stages, although this has not been proven effective in a controlled trial. When a patient who is several years post stroke seeks treatment, the authors tend to put them through an aggressive exercise program for swallowing muscles and then move to compensatory techniques if that fails. Crary and Bryant have reported success in the treatment of chronic dysphagia in brainstem stroke patients using electromyographic biofeedback to help guide swallow exercises.[60,61]

Multiple Sclerosis

Multiple sclerosis is a chronic, unpredictable, potentially debilitating inflammatory disease of varying severity. The affected sites are the myelin sheaths and the nerves they surround, potentially resulting in deficits in muscle coordination, strength, sensation, and vision. Multiple sclerosis affects approximately 300,000 persons in the United States and over 1 million worldwide, affecting women twice as often as men. Initial presentation is usually between the third and fifth decade, but the relapsing and remitting nature of the process can pose a challenge for diagnosis.[62]

As would be expected in a disease that affects muscle coordination, sensation, and strength, there is a high prevalence of oropharyngeal dysphagia. Over 30% of individuals with multiple sclerosis experience swallowing problems, a higher rate than previously assumed.[63] In addition, Terre-Boliart and colleagues[64] found through videofluoroscopic studies that up to 40% of these patients are silent aspirators.

Standard therapy has emphasized compensatory techniques in the past, but recent evidence suggests that exercise may have beneficial effects in this population.[65] As with other progressive diseases, this intervention is not a permanent remedy, and, eventually, dietary changes and careful feeding techniques are the mainstay of treatment. Complications from pneumonia are a common cause of morbidity and mortality in advanced multiple sclerosis; therefore, conservative and surgical therapies are aimed at preventing aspiration and resultant pneumonia.

AS COMPLICATIONS DEVELOP: SURGICAL OPTIONS
Recurrent Aspiration

When conservative measures to treat dysphagia and resultant aspiration have failed, surgical management becomes the final option to prevent life-threatening consequences of pneumonia and respiratory compromise. Tracheotomy is the universal treatment for patients with life-threatening aspiration; however, tracheotomy does not necessarily prevent aspiration. On the contrary, there can be an increased aspiration risk due to limitation of laryngeal elevation and anterosuperior excursion during swallowing.[66] Schonhofer and colleagues[67] demonstrated a 30% rate of aspiration in patients who underwent tracheotomy. This concern has come under criticism lately in a series of articles by Leder[34,68] who showed that, in many patients, there was no difference in their swallow with or without a tracheotomy. Rather, the underlying medical reason for needing the tracheostomy was the major cause of their aspiration. The main advantage of tracheotomy is that it permits more effective pulmonary toilet. Aggressive pulmonary toilet including suctioning must be maintained if tracheotomy is to be effective in preventing the consequences of aspiration.

When considering the multitude of permanent surgical options for aspiration, many factors must be taken into account, including comorbidities, the reason for aspiration, and the overall prognosis. **Table 1** lists the most common surgical options for patients with dysphagia with a brief discussion of each procedure.

Table 1
Surgical options for patients with dysphagia who are nonresponsive to conservative management

Procedure	Benefits	Indications	Contraindications
Tracheoesophageal diversion	Eliminates the larynx as a route of alimentation	When there is good prognosis for recovery of swallowing function	Disease of the upper trachea
Laryngotracheal separation	Preferred if tracheotomy is already present	Same as diversion	Same as diversion
Laryngeal suspension	Widens hypopharynx and keeps glottis closed during swallowing	Aspiration following supraglottic/hypopharyngectomy	Life-threatening aspiration
Glottic closure	Compensates for inadequate glottic closure	Aspiration secondary to vocal cord paralysis/atrophy	Patients without adequate pulmonary reserve
Vocal fold medialization	Preserves voice	Aspiration due to unilateral vocal cord paralysis	Laryngeal cancer, bilateral vocal cord paralysis, poor pulmonary status
Laryngeal closure	Glottis blocked off, forcing food down lateral pharynx	Inadequate glottic closure	Poor prognosis, as this is a reversible procedure
Total/partial cricoid resection	Larger opening into the hypopharynx aids with swallowing and smaller opening to the larynx reduces the risk of aspiration	When recovery of swallowing function is poor	Good prognosis for swallow recovery
Laryngectomy	Definitive treatment for aspiration	Reserved for severe neurologic impairment in nonverbal individuals or following resection of head and neck cancers, last resort	Anticipated neurologic/swallowing recovery or T1 and T2 laryngeal tumors

Tracheoesophageal diversion
First described by Lindeman,[68] this procedure provides for a complete separation of the digestive and respiratory organs. The procedure is performed by creating a complete transection of the trachea followed by an end-to-side tracheoesophageal anastomosis of the proximal portion of the trachea. The distal portion of the trachea is used as a tracheostomy. When a traditional high tracheotomy already exists in the patient, the tracheoesophageal anastomosis becomes more difficult, and a laryngotracheal separation may be a better option. Conversely, a modification by Krespi and colleagues[69] provides an option to address preexisting tracheotomy. The modification calls for resection of the proximal anterior tracheal cartilages and the inferior half of the cricoid cartilage to increase the mobility of the proximal trachea.

Laryngotracheal separation
In a follow-up article, Eisele and colleagues[70] described a modification to Lindeman's tracheoesophageal diversion which involves simply oversewing the proximal trachea, resulting in a blind pouch but at the same time removing the requirement for an esophageal anastomosis. This technique may be preferred over tracheoesophageal diversion when a tracheotomy already exists.

Laryngeal suspension
Calcaterra[71] first described the suspension of remnant laryngeal structures post supraglottic laryngectomy to supplement for the swallowing difficulties a patient would encounter after this procedure; however, Bocca and colleagues[72] actually reported suspension of the larynx remnant to the hyoid bone before Calcaterra. This procedure creates an enlarged opening to the hypopharynx and aids in keeping the glottis closed during swallowing by moving the larynx superiorly and interiorly while suspending the hyoid or thyroid lamina to mandible.

Glottic closure
First described by Montgomery,[73] glottic closure involves denuding and suturing of the true and false vocal cords. This procedure, by definition, will sacrifice the voice and causes irreparable damage to the vocal cords, essentially eliminating reversal as an option.

Vocal fold medialization
Please see references[74–79] and the article by Cohen and colleagues, elsewhere in this issue for a discussion on this topic.

Laryngeal closure
Supraglottic laryngeal closure, first reported by Habal and colleagues,[74] involves oversewing the epiglottis. It blocks off the entrance to the glottis, thereby redirecting food down the lateral pharyngeal channels. This option demands a tracheostomy but allows for potential postoperative phonation and reversibility. Since this original report, several modifications have been reported. Strome and colleagues[66] suggested severing supporting ligaments to decrease tension and reduce the possibility of dehiscence. Castellanos[75] created a second layer of closure by approximating the false vocal cords.

Total/partial cricoid resection
This procedure, first described by Krespi and colleagues,[76] involves removal of the posterior half of the cricoid lamina along with a cricopharyngeal and inferior constrictor myotomy. When done in the partial form, it allows for continued phonation providing that the recurrent laryngeal nerve and cricoarytenoid joints have not been damaged during the procedure.

Laryngectomy

First performed by Billroth in 1873,[77] laryngectomy is still regarded as the definitive treatment for intractible aspiration. Due to the irreversibility, loss of phonation, and cosmetic deformity, this procedure is used as a last resort after other modalities of treatment have failed. A popular modification to total laryngectomy has become narrow-field laryngectomy, which aims to preserve the hyoid, strap musculature, and the hypopharyngeal mucosa.

Sialorrhea

Sialorrhea, or hypersecretion, is actually a rare condition and is often a side effect of medications. The complaint of sialorrhea is most commonly a symptom of diminished oropharyngeal strength or control from neurologic disease. Aside from the cosmetic and functional disturbances that result from the normal output of 1.5 L of saliva produced daily,[78] uncontrolled salivation can be an additional cause of aspiration. Conservative therapies (oral motor training, behavioral therapy, and pharmacologic treatments) are generally effective when the problem is mild. When it is a significant handicap, patients often turn to surgery for resolution of symptoms. The otolaryngologist's role in the management of this disorder involves the following options.

Four-gland duct ligation

This procedure involves ligation of the two submandibular and two parotid ducts. The ligation can be accompanied by submandibular gland removal to eliminate the risk of abscess formation in the remaining glands. Martin and Conley[79] in a review of 31 patients who had undergone surgical treatment of sialorrhea noted a 68% rate of recurrence at 4 months postoperatively, indicating poor long-term control. In contrast, Shirley and colleagues[80] in a study of 21 patients who underwent four-duct ligation noted that 81% had improvement, with no regression during a 14-month follow-up period.

Salivary duct rerouting

Submandibular duct relocation, first described by Crysdale,[81] is a commonly performed procedure with excellent results. Some physicians advocate the additional removal of the sublingual glands at this time to decrease the incidence of ranula formation. McAloney and colleagues[82] were able to achieve good-to-excellent control in 16 of 21 patients with minimal side effects using rerouting with sublingual excision. De and colleagues[83] significantly reduced sialorrhea in 49 of their 56 cases; however, there were five cases of ranula formation in their series when they did not excise the sublingual glands. Parotid duct rerouting has fallen out of favor due to the significant morbidity that is often associated with the procedure.

Chorda tympani neurectomy

Transtympanic resection of the chorda tympani traditionally has a higher failure rate than the previously described procedures[84] owing to the regeneration of nerves. Gustatory deficits must also be taken into account when considering this option. Due to these adverse affects and low overall success rates combined with the knowledge that most sialorrhea is secondary and not a direct result of hypersecretion, this approach has fallen out of favor with most otolaryngologists.

Botulinum toxin

Botulinum toxin type A (Botox) has become an increasingly popular option for control of sialorrhea. Ellis and colleagues[85] reported an 80% efficacy rate in the treatment of sialorrhea attributable to head and neck carcinoma, neurodegenerative diseases, stroke, or idiopathic hypersalivation. They performed injections under ultrasound guidance with dosages ranging from 20 to 65 U. There is no agreed upon dosage to achieve adequate results. Lagalla and colleagues[86] have demonstrated efficacy via a double-blind, randomized, placebo-controlled study of 32 patient's with Parkinson's disease using 50 U into each parotid gland without the use of ultrasound with no adverse effects. Lipp and colleagues[87] were able to reduce saliva production by 50% with doses of 75 U into each parotid gland. In contrast to these studies, Su and colleagues[88] reported adequate control without side effects with only 40 U for the parotids and submandibular glands. Dogu and colleagues[89] in a study of 15 patients compared ultrasound-guided versus blind injection of Botox. There was a statistically significant decrease of secretions in the guided group, supporting the use of ultrasound.

Nutritional Issues

Enteral feeding

When considering alternative alimentation for patients whose oral intake is not optimal, one must consider the individual circumstance because different subgroups appear to respond differently to the type of intervention used. The safety and improved survival of using percutaneous endoscopic gastrostomy (PEG) tube feeding in patients with acute neurologic dysphagia from stroke or due to obstructing malignancy is well appreciated.[90] In a study of 415 cases of PEG placement for obstructing carcinomas of the upper digestive tract, Motsh and colleagues[91] found 81% patient compliance with the PEGs. This compliance along with the low complication rate led them to conclude that PEG placement was safe and effective for the long-term treatment of nutrition. This success has spawned its use for other debilitating diseases.

On the other hand, multiple studies of patients who have advanced dementia have shown that feeding tubes seldom are effective in improving nutrition, maintaining skin integrity by increased protein intake, preventing aspiration pneumonia, minimizing suffering, improving functional status, or extending life.[92] In a study of 361 consecutive patients with mixed medical diagnoses,[93] a mortality rate of 28% at 30 days was found for all patients requiring gastrostomy feeding. Patients with dementia had an even worse prognosis, with 54% having died at 1 month and 90% at 1 year. Survival outcomes after PEG insertion are poor for patients over 80 years of age or with diabetes, whereas better outcomes are found in demented patients aged less than 80 years.[94] Patients need to be treated on an individual basis and have all of their risk factors taken into consideration rather than applying blanket treatment to various subgroups.

The efficacy of PEG placement in patients with ALS is equivocal. When oral food intake becomes intolerable because of frequent choking or excess weight loss, a PEG tube should be seriously considered.[95,96] Guidelines of the American Academy of Neurology recommend that the PEG tube be placed before forced vital capacity (FVC) drops below 50% because of increased risks of respiratory complications during and immediately after the PEG procedure.[97] In patients with a FVC less than 50%, PEG placement should be done only after institution of noninvasive ventilation.[98] A recent Cochrane review found evidence in favor of placing a PEG tube in bulbar onset ALS patients but could not unequivocally recommend enteral feeding in limb onset patients.[99] In the authors' clinics, we have found that early education of the benefits of PEG placement has helped bulbar onset patients accept it before they are in crisis and need it emergently. In fact, they generally report better quality of life after having the PEG because of improved nutritional status, energy level, and time to devote to other activities. We do not recommend a PEG for all limb onset patients, because some patients experience significant respiratory symptoms before dysphagia emerges and may not ever reach the point where a PEG is necessary before their demise from respiratory failure. This issue is a very personal and individual one that the health care provider, patient, and family need to discuss thoroughly to make the best decision.

WHEN PALLIATIVE CARE IS NEEDED

Throughout the course of a disease, practitioners should perform follow-up with clinical and instrumental swallowing studies to evaluate the patient's swallowing ability along with their nutrition, health status, and the patient's and family's desires. With this information, the clinician can determine the optimum course of treatment, including termination of treatment that is no longer viable. The clinician must be cognizant of the following signs and symptoms of unremitting dysphagia or increased risk for aspiration when choosing to persist in or desist from traditional therapeutic interventions:

1. Patient and family reports of limited oral intake, persistent throat clearing or coughing during eating, and disrupted breathing and sleeping
2. Associated risk factors or symptoms such as general weakness and mental status changes
3. Changes in medical diagnosis such as recent stroke or thyroid disease
4. Introduction of new medications
5. Recurrent aspiration pneumonias
6. Significant weight loss of greater than 5% to 10% or recurrent episodes of dehydration requiring enteral methods of feeding
7. Laryngoscopic evidence of excessive saliva pooled in the larynx and inability of the patient to protect the airway or swallow
8. Radiologic demonstration of lack of a functional swallow

Despite the best efforts of surgeons and speech pathologists, many patients are left with persistent intractable dysphagia. For these patients, oral intake is severely limited or nonexistent and airway protection is reduced, placing them at risk for nutritional insufficiency, dehydration, malnutrition, and aspiration pneumonia. A permanent alternate means of nutrition is often indicated. Tracheotomy for direct airway access and suctioning of aspirated secretions may be necessary, or other more permanent surgical interventions may be considered.

As discussed previously, enteral feeding is not a panacea, and the decision to resort to tube feeding must be made with careful consideration of the patient's prognosis, wishes, and competence because this decision will affect their quality of life. Nearly every social activity we engage in includes eating and sometimes takes place entirely around a dining table. Patients with an inability to eat orally may become socially isolated. Conversely, patients who constantly cough and choke may avoid eating situations as well. Anecdotal reports of patients in nursing homes tell us of residents whose dysphagia is severe enough to result in placement of a feeding tube. This "final solution" to their dysphagia can have significant and adverse consequences and trigger a downward spiral. It begins with their being excluded from meals in the dining room, leading to less social interaction with other residents, followed by spending more time in bed, and ending in a "failure to thrive" and imminent death. Inserting a feeding tube appears to hasten mortality in some people when the intent was originally to improve their health status.

These anecdotes point out how serious and complicated the issue can be when a patient has severe chronic dysphagia. The only tenable solution is to involve the patient and the family in the decision making. The clinician can contribute to this process by providing an explanation of what is wrong with the patient's swallow and what, if anything, may improve it. This discussion should be followed by comprehensive information regarding the advantages and disadvantages of tube feeding, a discussion of how aspiration pneumonia develops, and the importance of good nutrition. Armed with this information, it is hoped that the patient and family will make the best decision. Whenever possible, a combination of foods or liquids by mouth combined with enteral feeding for nutrition results in the "best of both worlds." Oral intake, even if just water sips, may reduce drooling or aspiration of secretions and will help with the perception of thirst or dry mouth.

Regardless of whether the decision is made to convert to complete tube feeding, to continue oral feeding, or to engage in some combination of both, other risk factors for pneumonia in addition to dysphagia should be considered by the clinician and addressed in treatment. These factors include safe and careful feeding or self-feeding (eg, safe posture, slow small bolus sizes), strict oral hygiene measures (brushing the teeth several times per day), aggressive pulmonary toilet, hygienic suctioning protocols, and keeping the patient as active as possible and upright during the day. In addition, reflux precautions at night are imperative. In studies performed by Langmore and colleagues,[100,101] these risk factors were found to be stronger predictors of aspiration pneumonia than the presence of dysphagia and aspiration in a group of inpatients, outpatients, and nursing home patients. If these risk factors are attended to, the odds of the patient contracting aspiration pneumonia may be diminished. Although some may say "pneumonia is the friend of the elderly," we believe it is often premature and never a comfortable way to die. We owe it to our patients to keep them as healthy and comfortable as possible.

FUTURE DIRECTIONS: NEW THERAPIES FOR DYSPHAGIA
Electrical Stimulation

Recently, a new therapy has been introduced for oropharyngeal dysphagia called e-stim, Vital Stim, or Neuromuscular Electrical Stimulation (NMES). Modeled after a system of therapy used in rehabilitation medicine, this modality transmits low voltage current via skin surface electrodes, triggering a nerve to fire and inducing muscular contraction. NMES works by improving the nerve-muscle interaction and contractile properties of the muscle and priming the afferent loop of the motor system. NMES is a rehabilitation modality that has shown clear benefits for improving aberrant extremity motor function.[102,103] The strongest clinical evidence for benefit is a recent meta-analysis of randomized controlled trials showing that electromyographic triggered NMES improves arm, hand, and finger function after stroke.[104] To date, four published articles have reported outcomes of this therapy with patients having dysphagia.[104–107] The publications are encouraging, but most of them were uncontrolled, using patients with a variety of medical diagnoses.

The author and her colleagues at Boston University Medical Center have initiated a multicenter, National Institutes of Health (NIH) funded randomized clinical trial to determine whether there is an objective benefit to swallowing function from a therapy program using NMES in post-radiated head and neck cancer patients with dysphagia. This protocol is aimed at a group of patients with early dysphagia due to the adverse effects of radiotherapy. Because of the continuing fibrosis that results from radiotherapy, clinical experience has shown that the dysphagia often becomes chronic and worsens over time if not treated effectively in the early stages. NMES is a treatment that it is hoped will prevent chronic dysphagia.

Neural Implants

Ludlow and colleagues at the NIH are currently conducting a phase II clinical study to evaluate an implanted neuroprosthesis for dysphagia. They are studying patients with evidence of severe and chronic pharyngeal phase dysphagia from stroke or chronic neurologic disease. The goal is to determine whether the implanted neuroprosthesis will improve swallowing in chronic pharyngeal dysphagia to the point where the patient can eat orally again without aspirating. The neuroprosthesis, under patient control, provides intramuscular stimulation to as many as eight hyolaryngeal muscles. This study is probably the most dramatic surgical treatment for dysphagia ever proposed. If successful, it will provide some hope to those afflicted with chronic life-threatening dysphagia.[108,109]

SUMMARY

This article has attempted to cover the issues faced by patients, caretakers, and clinicians when dysphagia is a chronic and serious complication of an underlying disease. Palliative care for this problem cannot be passive. It requires consultation, compassion, and collaborative decision making to help persons face end of life with dignity and maximum quality of life. If drooling, choking, and coughing can be minimized while meeting a patient's need for thirst and hunger, our goals will have been met.

REFERENCES

1. Howden CW. Management of acid-related disorders in patients with dysphagia. Am J Med 2004;117(5A):44–8.
2. Domench E, Kelly J. Swallowing disorders. Med Clin North Am 1999;83(1): 97–113.
3. Marik PE, Kaplan D. Aspiration pneumonia and dysphagia in the elderly. Chest 2003;124(1):328–36.
4. Logemann J, Rademaker A, Pauloski B, et al. Effects of postural change on aspiration in head and neck surgical patients. Otolaryngol Head Neck Surg 1994; 110:222–7.
5. Lazarus C, Logemann J, Rademaker A, et al. Effects of bolus volume, viscosity, and repeated swallows in nonstroke subjects and stroke patients. Arch Phys Med Rehabil 1993;74(10):1066–70.
6. Lazarus C. Effects of radiation therapy and voluntary maneuvers on swallow functioning in head and neck cancer patients. Clin Comm Disord 1993;3:11–20.
7. Lazarus C, Logemann J, Song C, et al. Effects of voluntary maneuvers on tongue base function for swallowing. Folia Phoniatr Logop 2002;54:171–6.
8. Veis S, Logemann J, Colangelo L. Effects of three techniques on maximum posterior movement of the tongue base. Dysphagia 2000;15:142–5.
9. Robbins J, Kay SA, Gangnon RE, et al. The effects of lingual exercise in stroke patients with dysphagia. Arch Phys Med Rehabil 2007;88(2):150.
10. Shaker R, Easterling C, Kern M, et al. Rehabilitation of swallowing by exercise in tube-fed patients with pharyngeal dysphagia secondary to abnormal UES opening. Gastroenterology 2002;122(5):1314–21.
11. Lazarus C. Tongue strength and exercise in healthy individuals and in head and neck cancer patients. Semin Spech Lang 2006;27(4):260–7.
12. Logemann JA, Kahrilas PJ. Relearning to swallow after stroke: application of maneuvers and indirect biofeedback. A case study. Neurology 1990;40:1136–8.

13. Logemann JA, Pauloski BR, Colangelo L, et al. Effects of a sour bolus on oropharyngeal swallowing measures in patients with neurogenic dysphagia. J Speech Hear Res 1995;38:556–63.
14. Logemann JA, Pauloski BR, Rademaker AW, et al. Super-supraglottic swallow in irradiated head and neck cancer patients. Head Neck 1997;19:535–40.
15. Mittal B, Pauloski B, Haraf D, et al. Swallowing dysfunction—preventative and rehabilitation strategies in patients with head-and-neck cancers treated with surgery, radiotherapy, and chemotherapy: a critical review. Int J Radiat Oncol Biol Phys 2003;57(5):1219–30.
16. Pauloski B, Logemann J, Rademaker A, et al. Speech and swallowing functions after anterior tongue and floor-of-mouth resection with distal flap reconstruction. J Speech Hear Res 1993;36:267–76.
17. Hirano M, Kuroiwa Y, Tanaka S, et al. Dysphagia following various degrees of surgical resection for oral cancer. Ann Otol Rhinol Laryngol 1992;101:138–41.
18. Logemann J, Pauloski B, Rademaker A, et al. Speech and swallowing function after tonsil/base-of-tongue resection with primary closure. J Speech Hear Res 1993;36:918–26.
19. Logemann J, Bytall D. Swallowing disorders in three types of head and neck surgical patients. Cancer 1979;81:469–78.
20. Zuydam A, Rogers S, Brown J, et al. Swallowing rehabilitation after oropharyngeal resection for squamous cell carcinoma. Br J Oral Maxillofac Surg 2000;38:513–8.
21. Marchese-Ragona R, De Grandis D, Restivo D, et al. Recovery of swallowing disorders in patients undergoing supracricoid laryngectomy with botulinum toxin therapy. Ann Otol Rhinol Laryngol 2003;112(3):258–63.
22. Induction chemotherapy plus radiation compared with surgery plus radiation in patients with advanced laryngeal cancer. The Department of Veterans Affairs Laryngeal Cancer Study Group. N Engl J Med 1991;324:1685–90.
23. Forastiere A, Goepfert H, Maor M, et al. Concurrent chemotherapy and radiotherapy for organ preservation in advanced laryngeal cancer. N Engl J Med 2003;349:2091–8.
24. Henk J. Controlled trials of synchronous chemotherapy with radiotherapy in head and neck cancer: overview of radiation morbidity. Clin Oncol (R Coll Radiol) 1997;9:308–12.
25. Delaney G, Fisher R, Smee R, et al. Split-course accelerated therapy in head-and-neck cancer: an analysis of toxicity. Int J Radiat Oncol Biol Phys 1995;32:763–8.
26. Cooper J, Fu K, Marks J, et al. Late effects of radiation therapy in head and neck region. Int J Radiat Oncol Biol Phys 1995;31:1141–64.
27. Pauloski B, Logemann J. Impact of tongue-base and posterior-pharyngeal wall biomechanics on pharyngeal clearance in irradiated post-surgical oral and oropharyngeal cancer patients. Head Neck 2000;22:120–31.
28. Nguyen N, Moltz C, Frank C, et al. Aspiration rate following nonsurgical therapy for laryngeal cancer. J Otorhinlaryngol Relat Spec 2007;69(2):116–20.
29. Lazarus C, Logemann J, Pauloski B, et al. Swallowing disorders in head and neck cancer patients treated with radiotherapy and adjuvant chemotherapy. Laryngoscope 1996;106:1157–66.
30. Logemann J, Rademaker A, Pauloski B, et al. Site of disease and treatment protocol as correlates of swallowing function in patients with head and neck cancer treated with chemoradiation. Head Neck 2006;28(1):64–73.

31. Tandan R, Bradley WG. Amyotrophic lateral sclerosis. Part 1. Clinical features, pathology, and ethical issues in management. Ann Neurol 1985;18:271–80.
32. Strand E, Miller R, Yorkston K, et al. Management of oral-pharyngeal symptoms in amyotrophic lateral sclerosis. Dysphagia 1996;11:129–39.
33. Mulder DS. The diagnosis and treatment of amyotrophic lateral sclerosis. Boston: Houghton Mifflin; 1980.
34. Leder SB, Novella S, Patwa H. Use of fiberoptic endoscopic evaluation of swallowing in patients with amyotropic lateral sclerosis. Dysphagia 2004;19(3): 177–81.
35. Lomen-Hoerth C, MJ, Langmore S, et al. Characterization of amyotrophic lateral sclerosis and frontotemporal dementia. Dement Geriatr Cogn Disord 2004;17(4): 337–41.
36. Mayo Clinic Research Center. Available at: http://cancercenter.mayo.edu/mayo/research/parkinsons/. Accessed January 9, 2008.
37. Edwards L, Quigley E, Pffeifer R. Gastrointestinal dysfunction in Parkinson's disease, frequency and pathophysiology. Neurology 1992;42:726–32.
38. Potulska A, Friedman A, Królicki L, et al. Swallowing disorders in Parkinson's disease. Parkinsonism Relat Disord 2003;9(6):349–53.
39. Nagaya M, Kachi T, Yamada T. Effect of swallowing training on swallowing disorders in Parkinson's disease. Scand J Rehabil Med 2000;32(1):11–5.
40. Diamond A, Jankovic J. Treatment of advanced Parkinson's disease. Expert Rev Neurother 2006;6(8):1181–97.
41. Bushmann M, Dobmeyer SM, Leeker L, et al. Swallowing abnormalities and their response to treatment in Parkinson's disease. Neurology 1989;39(10):1309–14.
42. Centers for Disease Control and Prevention. Available at: www.cdc.gov. Accessed January 9, 2008.
43. Chen J-H, Lamberg JL, Chen Y-C, et al. Occurrence and treatment of suspected pneumonia in long-term care residents dying with advanced dementia. JAGS 54:290–5.
44. Litvan I, Mangone CA, McKee A, et al. Natural history of progressive supranuclear palsy (Steele-Richardson-Olszewski syndrome) and clinical predictors of survival: a clinicopathological study. J Neuro Neurosurg Psych 1996;61:615–20.
45. Feinberg MJ, Ekberg O, Segall L, et al. Deglutition in elderly patients with dementia: findings of videofluorographic evaluation and impact on staging and management. Radiology 1992;183(3):811–4.
46. Priefer BA, Robbins J. Eating changes in mild-stage Alzheimer's disease: a pilot study. Dysphagia 1997;12(4):212–21.
47. Langmore S, Olney R, Lomen-Hoerth C, et al. Dysphagia in patients with frontotemporal lobar dementia. Arch Neurol 2007;64(1):58–62.
48. National Stroke Association. Stroke fact sheet. Available at: http://www.stroke.org/site/DocServer/STROKE_101_Fact_Sheet.pdf?docID=4541. Accessed January 9, 2008.
49. National Institute of Health: Heart Lung and Blood Institute. Available at: http://www.nhlbi.nih.gov/. Accessed January 9, 2008.
50. Glickenstein GW, Stein J, Ambrosi D, et al. Predictors of survival after severe dysphagic stroke. J Neurol 2005;252(12):1510–6.
51. Smithard DG, O'Neill PA, England RE, et al. The natural history of dysphagia following a stroke [see comment]. Dysphagia 1997;12(4):188–93.
52. Wade DT, Langton-Hewer R. Motor loss and swallowing difficulty after stroke: frequency, recovery, and prognosis. Acta Neurol Scand 1987;76:50–4.

53. Logemann JA. Evaluation and treatment of swallowing disorders. 2nd edition. Austin (TX): Pro-Ed; 1997.
54. Robbins J, Levine RL, Maser A, et al. Swallowing after unilateral stroke of the cerebral cortex. Arch Phys Med Rehabil 1993;74(12):1295–300.
55. Daniels SK, Foundas AL. Lesion localization in acute stroke patients with risk of aspiration. J Neuroimaging 1999;9(2):91–8.
56. Daniels SK. Swallowing apraxia: a disorder of the praxis system? Dysphagia 2000;15:159–66.
57. Teasell R, Foley N, Fisher J, et al. The incidence, management, and complications of dysphagia in patients with medullary strokes admitted to a rehabilitation unit. Dysphagia 2002;17(2):115–20.
58. Hyanghee K, Chung C-S, Kwang-Ho L, et al. Aspiration subsequent to a pure medullary infarction: lesion sites, clinical variables, and outcome. Arch Neurol 2000;57(4):478–83.
59. Meng NH, Wang TG, Lien IN. Dysphagia in patients with brainstem stroke: incidence and outcome. Am J Phys Med Rehab 2000;79(2):170–5.
60. Crary MA, Carnaby GD, Groher ME. Biomechanical correlates of surface electromyography signals obtained during swallowing by healthy adults. J Speech Lang Hear Res 2006;49:186–93.
61. Bryant M. Biofeedback in the treatment of a selected dysphagic patient. Dysphagia 1991;6:140–4.
62. Mayo Clinic. Available at: http://www.mayoclinic.com/health/multiple-sclerosis/DS00188. Accessed January 9, 2008.
63. Prosiegel M, Schelling A, Wagner-Sonntag E. Dysphagia and multiple sclerosis. Int MS J 2004;11(1):22–31.
64. Terre-Boliart R, Orient-Lopez F, Guevera-Espinosa D, et al. Oropharyngeal dysphagia in patients with multiple sclerosis. Rev Neurol 2004;39(8):707–10.
65. Bjarnadottir OH, Reynisdottir K, Olafsson E. Multiple sclerosis and brief moderate exercise: a randomised study. Mult Scler 2007;13(6):776–82.
66. Strome M, Shapiro J. Aspiration. In: Fried MP, editor. The larynx: a multidisciplinary approach. 2nd edition. St Louis (MO): Mosby-Year Book; 1996. p. 358.
67. Schonhofer B, Barchfeld T, Haidl P, et al. Scintigraphy for evaluating early aspiration after oral feeding in patients receiving prolonged ventilation via tracheostomy. Intensive Care Med 1999;25(3):311–4.
68. Lindeman RC. Diverting the paralyzed larynx: a reversible procedure for intractable aspiration. Laryngoscope 1975;85(1):157–80.
69. Krespi YP, Quatela VC, Sisson GA, et al. Modified tracheoesophageal diversion for chronic aspiration. Laryngoscope 1984;94(10):1298–301.
70. Eisele DW, Yarington CT Jr, Lindeman RC. Indications for the tracheoesophageal diversion procedure and the laryngotracheal separation procedure. Ann Otol Rhinol Laryngol 1988;97(5 Pt 1):471–572.
71. Calcaterra TC. Laryngeal suspension after supraglottic laryngectomy. Arch Otolaryngol 1971;94(4):306–9.
72. Bocca E, Pignataro O, Mosciaro O. Supraglottic surgery of the larynx. Ann Otol Rhinol Laryngol 1968;77:1005–126.
73. Montgomery WW. Surgery to prevent aspiration. Arch Otolaryngol 1975;101(11):679–80.
74. Habal MB, Murray JE. Surgical treatment of life-endangering chronic aspiration pneumonia: use of an epiglottic flap to the arytenoids. Plast Reconstr Surg 1972;49(3):305–11.

75. Castellanos PF. Method and clinical results of a new transthyrotomy closure of the supraglottic larynx for the treatment of intractable aspiration. Ann Otol Rhinol Laryngol 1997;106(6):451–60.

76. Krespi YP, Pelzer HJ, Sisson GA. Management of chronic aspiration by subtotal and submucosal cricoid resection. Ann Otol Rhinol Laryngol 1985;94(6 Pt 1): 580–3.

77. Chas M, Steinberg BJ, et al. Surgery of the larynx. Philadelphia: WB Saunders; 1985. p. 322.

78. Lee KJ. Essential otolaryngology: head and neck surgery. East Norwalk, CT: Appleton & Lange; 1999. p. 459.

79. Martin TJ, Conley SF. Long-term efficacy of intraoral surgery for sialorrhea. Otolaryngol Head Neck Surg 2007;137(1):54–8.

80. Shirley WP, Hill JS, Woolley AL, et al. Success and complications of four-duct ligation for Sialorrhea. Int J Pediatr Otorhinolaryngol 2003;67(1):1–6.

81. Crysdale WS, White A. Submandibular duct relocation for drooling: a 10-year experience with 194 patients. Otolaryngol Head Neck Surg 1989;101:87–92.

82. McAloney N, Kerawala CJ, Stassen LF. Management of drooling by transposition of the submandibular ducts and excision of the sublingual glands. J Ir Dent Assoc 2005;51(3):126–31.

83. De M, Adair R, Golchin K, et al. Outcomes of submandibular duct relocation: a 15-year experience. J Laryngol Otol 2003;117(10):821–3.

84. Parisier SC, Blitzer A, Binder WJ, et al. Tympanic neurectomy and chorda tympanectomy for the control of drooling. Arch Otolaryngol 1978;104:273–7.

85. Ellies M, Gottstein U, Rohrbach-Volland S, et al. Reduction of salivary flow with botulinum toxin: extended report on 33 patients with drooling, salivary fistulas, and sialadenitis. Laryngoscope 2004;114(10):1856–60.

86. Lagalla G, Millevolte M, Capecci M, et al. Botulinum toxin type A for drooling in Parkinson's disease: a double-blind, randomized, placebo-controlled study. Mov Disord 2006;21(5):704–7.

87. Lipp A, Trottenberg T, Schink T, et al. A randomized trial of botulinum toxin A for the treatment of drooling. Neurology 2003;61:1279–81.

88. Su CS, Lan MY, Liu JS, et al. Botulinum toxin type A treatment for parkinsonian patients with moderate to severe sialorrhea. Acta Neurol Taiwan 2006;15(3): 170–6.

89. Dogu O, Apaydin D, Sevim S, et al. Ultrasound-guided versus 'blind' intraparotid injections of botulinum toxin A for the treatment of sialorrhoea in patients with Parkinson's disease. Clin Neurol Neurosurg 2004;106(2):93–6.

90. James A, Kapur K, Hawthorne AB. Long-term outcome of percutaneous endoscopic gastrostomy feeding in patients with dysphagic stroke. Age Ageing 1998;27:671–6.

91. Motsch C, Hackelsberger A, Nebelung K. Percutaneous endoscopic gastrostomy in patients with ENT tumors. HNO 1998;46(11):925–31.

92. Cervo FA, Bryan L, Farber S. To PEG or not to PEG: a review of evidence for placing feeding tubes in advanced dementia and the decision-making process. Geriatrics 2006;61(6):30–5.

93. Sanders DS, Carter MJ, D'Silva J, et al. Survival analysis in percutaneous endoscopic gastrostomy feeding: a worse outcome in patients with dementia. Am J Gastroenterol 2000;95(6):1472–5.

94. Rimon E, Kagansy N, Levy S. Percutaneous endoscopic gastrostomy: evidence of different prognosis in various patient subgroups. Age Ageing 2005;34:353–7.

95. Kasarskis EJ, et al. A retrospective study of percutaneous endoscopic gastrostomy in ALS patients during the BDNF and CNTF trials. J Neurol Sci 1999; 169:118–25.
96. Andersen PM, Borasio GD, Dengler R, et al. EFNS Task Force on Diagnosis and Management of Amyotrophic Lateral Sclerosis. EFNS task force on management of amyotrophic lateral sclerosis: guidelines for diagnosing and clinical care of patients and relatives. Eur J Neurol 2005;12(12):921–38.
97. Miller RG, Rosenberg JA, Gelinas DF, et al. Practice parameter: the care of the patient with amyotrophic lateral sclerosis (an evidence-based review). Report of the Quality Standards Subcommittee of the American Academy of Neurology: ALS Practice Parameters Task Force. Neurology 1999;52(7):1311–23.
98. Gregory S, Siderowf A, Golaszewski AL, et al. Gastrostomy insertion in ALS patients with low vital capacity: respiratory support and survival. Neurology 2002;58:485–7.
99. Langmore SE, Kasanskis E, Manca ML, et al. Enteral tube feeding for amyotrophic lateral sclerosis/motor neuron disease. Cochrane Database Syst Rev 2006; 4: CD004030.
100. Langmore SE, Terpenning MS, Schork A, et al. Predictors of aspiration pneumonia: how important is dysphagia? Dysphagia 1998;13(2):69–81.
101. Langmore SE, Skarupski KA, Park PS, et al. Predictors of aspiration pneumonia in nursing home residents. Dysphagia 2002;17(4):298–307.
102. Kimberley T, Lewis S, Auerbach E, et al. Electrical stimulation driving functional improvements and cortical changes in subjects with stroke. Exp Brain Res 2004; 154:450–60.
103. Cauraugh J, Light K, Kim S, et al. Chronic motor dysfunction after stroke: recovering wrist and finger extension by electromyography-triggered neuromuscular stimulation. Stroke 2000;30:1360–4.
104. Bolton D, Cauraugh J, Hausenblas H. Electromyogram-triggered neuromuscular stimulation and stroke motor recover of arm/hand functions: a meta-analysis. J Neuro Sci 2004;223:121–7.
105. Freed M, Freed L, Chatburn R, et al. Electrical stimulation for swallowing disorders caused by stroke. Respir Care 2001;46(5):466–74.
106. Leelamanit V, Limsakul C, Geater A. Synchronized electrical stimulation in treating pharyngeal dysphagia. Laryngoscope 2002;112:2204–10.
107. Blumenfeld L, Hahn Y, LePage A, et al. Transcutaneous electrical stimulation versus traditional dysphagia therapy: a nonconcurrent cohort study. Otolaryngol Head Neck Surg 2006;135:754–7.
108. Ludlow CL, Humbert K, Saxon K, et al. Effects of surface electrical stimulation both at rest and during swallowing in chronic pharyngeal dysphagia. Dysphagia 2006;1–10.
109. National Institutes of Health. Registered clinical trials. Available at: http://clinicaltrials. gov/ct/show/NCT00376506?order=1. Accessed January 9, 2008.

Palliative Treatment of Dysphonia and Dysarthria

Seth M. Cohen, MD, MPH[a], Alphi Elackattu, MD[b], J. Pieter Noordzij, MD[b],*,
Michael J. Walsh, MA[b], Susan E. Langmore, PhD[b]

KEYWORDS

- Palliative • Dysphonia • Dysarthria • Hoarseness
- Laryngectomy

Voice disorders can have a drastic impact on the quality of life (QOL) of patients because they adversely affect one of the most basic of facilities: communication.[1,2] Speech is a complex action requiring precise motor control of the upper digestive and respiratory tracts. Speech production relies on several highly integrated factors that Kantner and West[3] divided into (1) respiration, (2) phonation, (3) resonation, (4) articulation, and (5) neurologic integration. Speech begins with respiration, which provides power during exhalation to vibrate the vocal cords, called "phonation," producing a complex tone. This tone is modified by the resonators: the pharyngeal, oral, and nasal cavities. It is then shaped by the movement of the tongue, soft palate, teeth, and lips during articulation to arrive at the end result, which is fully formed speech.[4]

Voice disorders can be grouped into two main classes depending on the level of the defect: dysarthria and dysphonia. Dysarthria is caused by neurologic damage to the motor components of speech, which may involve any or all of the speech processes, including respiration, phonation, articulation, resonance, and prosody. Dysphonia refers to disordered sound production at the level of the larynx, classically seen as hoarseness. It may have a neurologic, structural, or functional etiology. It is important not to confuse either of these terms with aphasia, which is a disorder of language caused by neurologic damage. Voice disorders have varying lengths of duration and treatment options depending on the underlying etiology.

THERAPEUTIC OPTIONS

Standard voice therapy for dysphonia aims to rehabilitate the voice whenever possible, meaning to restore normal function. When that is not possible because of the underlying pathology, the aim is to achieve a voice that is as normal as possible, as

[a] Division of Otolaryngology, Head and Neck Surgery, Duke University, Durham, NC, USA
[b] Department of Otolaryngology, Head and Neck Surgery, Boston University Medical Center, 820 Harrison Avenue, FGH Building, 4th Floor, Boston, MA 02118, USA
* Corresponding author.
E-mail address: noordzij@bu.edu (J.P. Noordzij).

Otolaryngol Clin N Am 42 (2009) 107–121
doi:10.1016/j.otc.2008.09.010
0030-6665/08/$ – see front matter © 2009 Elsevier Inc. All rights reserved.

oto.theclinics.com

pleasant as possible, and achieved with as least effort as possible. Methods of voice therapy can be categorized in several different ways. For dysphonia where the voice is hypophonic, the clinician aims to energize the voice, or make it stronger, louder, and with greater prosodic range (eg, Lee Silverman Voice Treatment, developed by Ramig and coworkers).[5] If the voice is hyperphonic (strained, harsh, or tight), the clinician focuses on relaxing the voice quality and may also focus on altering pitch and intonation (eg, stretch and flow phonation[6] or laryngeal massage).[7,8] Sometimes, the focus in voice therapy is simply to normalize the voice by focusing on optimal breathing and resonance.[9,10]

When standard treatments with voice therapy have been exhausted, patients may turn to augmentative alternative communication (AAC) modalities to maintain their ability to communicate. This approach ranges from using visual or gestural cues to using more complicated computer-based technology that "speaks" for the patient to help communicate. As a confounder, the very disease process that has stripped the patient of their vocal abilities may also limit the options one has for alternative means of communication. Early and appropriate referral to determine AAC options is the most important intervention that needs to occur.

Surgery is the final option that can palliate the dysphonic patient, although not necessarily cure the underlying condition. Examples include placing a tracheoesophageal (TE) prosthesis and augmenting an atrophic vocal fold with collagen. In each of these two examples the underlying medical condition is not cured.

SPECIFIC DISEASES
Amyotrophic Lateral Sclerosis

Bulbar amyotrophic lateral sclerosis (ALS) is known to present with speech problems and has a more severe disease progression overall. Bulbar involvement usually manifests initially with both upper motor neuron (UMN) and lower motor neuron (LMN) involvement. It can present initially, however, as only affecting LMN (progressive bulbar palsy) or UMN (primary lateral sclerosis). Eventually, both upper and lower neurons are affected if the disease is truly ALS.

LMN involvement may present initially by affecting any cranial nerve unilaterally or bilaterally, but eventually it affects all of them bilaterally. LMN damage presents as weakness and atrophy, and increased fatigue. The resting tone is hypotonic. Voice becomes breathy and weak when the vagus nerve is damaged and resonance becomes hypernasal when the muscles and nerves innervating the soft palate are affected. Respiratory weakness (especially from damage to the diaphragm by the phrenic nerve) contributes to a soft voice because of reduced respiratory support for speech. Speech therapy early on may emphasize clear exaggerated articulation and compensatory techniques to help the voice be heard because increased effort may be counterproductive. Voice amplifiers may also be helpful in this regard.

UMN involvement generally affects all the cranial nerves innervating the speech and voice systems. UMN damage causes slowness, loss of precise movements, hypertonicity, and central fatigue. The voice is tight, hoarse, and strained. Velopharyngeal closure may be complete but slow to move; hypernasality is inconsistent. Respiratory support is reduced because of rigidity, but not weakness, and the voice is adequately loud. Rapid vocal changes are not possible; pitch and loudness adversely affect prosody and are perceived as monotone and monoloudness. Voice therapy can help patients in the early changes by teaching volitional relaxation of laryngeal muscles and better breath support and control for speech.

The use of AAC in this population becomes increasingly valuable if the patient chooses invasive ventilation to prolong his or her life. A review by Ball and coworkers[11] showed that ALS patients often use their AAC within weeks of their death, presumably aiding communication at this critical time. Patients with primary bulbar ALS used their AAC technology an average of 24.9 months, whereas those with spinal ALS used their AAC technology for an average of 31.1 months. In this population, it has been recommended[12] that patients be referred for AAC when their spoken reading rate slows to 100 to 125 words per minute (normal is 190 words per minute) or if they must repeat frequently to be understood. Eventually, the dysarthria of ALS may lead to anarthria and AAC becomes necessary for communication. Although most of the computerized systems now include a synthetic voice, newer voices are being developed that sound more natural and are easier for listeners to accept.[13]

When they are no longer able to type on a keyboard to communicate, patients have a multitude of options including computers that are accessed by dynamic touch screens, and head-tracking and eye-tracking technologies. AAC may enable even quadriplegic patients to communicate effectively.[14] First attempts at directly exploiting brain electric currents to control computers have shown encouraging results. Kubler and colleagues[15] have reported that they were able to help four people severely disabled by ALS to learn to operate a brain-computer interface with electroencephalogram rhythms recorded over the sensorimotor cortex. At this stage, however, the communication systems are not practically functional.

For surgical options in palliating ALS, Esposito and colleagues[16] reviewed the efficacy of a palatal lift or augmentation prosthesis to improve speech in 25 ALS patients. They were able to demonstrate that 84% treated with a palatal lift demonstrated improvement in their dysarthria, specifically in reduction of hypernasality, and 19 (76%) of these patients benefited at least moderately for 6 months. Of the 10 patients treated with a combination palatal lift and augmentation prosthesis, 6 (60%) demonstrated improvement in articulation.[16]

Parkinson's Disease

Disorders of voice and speech within this population is estimated to be 70% to 85%, with greater than 30% of these patients finding it to be the most disabling part of the disorder.[17] Severity is often directly related to the other physical symptoms seen. The underlying physiologic problems include akinesia, bradykinesia, rigidity, and tremor. Parkinsonian speech is classically monopitch, of reduced vocal intensity, hoarse, harsh or breathy voice in quality, with articulatory imprecision, and of a variable rate with short rushes of speech punctuated by inappropriate silence.[18] Fluorographic studies have demonstrated the most common progression of vocal tract symptoms, which begins with laryngeal dysfunction, followed by alterations in lingual and subsequently labial functions.[19] In a study by Perez and colleagues,[20] vocal tremor was found in 55% of Parkinson's patients.

Despite the high incidence of speech and voice impairment, studies suggest that only 3% to 4% of people with Parkinson's disease (PD) receive speech treatment.[21] Voice therapy is of great benefit to Parkinson's patients in the early and mid stages. A well-researched program shown to be effective and efficacious is the Lee Silverman Voice Treatment, developed by Ramig and coworkers.[5] This therapy teaches the patient to self-cue him or herself to speak loudly. When speaking loudly, other aspects of voice and speech generally improve, so the final result is a louder, better intoned voice with better breath support and clearer articulation.

In the early to middle stages of speech dysfunction, PD patients are managed with rehabilitative voice therapy, and sometimes with amplifiers. In later stages, behavioral or environmental techniques may be useful. Alphabet supplementation,[22] where the patient points to the first letter of each word as he or she says it, is designed to control speech rates and provide the listener with additional visual cues. Techniques using changes to the patients' environment can be used to facilitate communication.[23] In a small portion of PD patients, all speech may be lost. Because of the overall motor control impairment and the frequent cognitive impairment in late disease, complex AAC interventions are difficult to institute. These patients typically do best with letter-by-letter typing with print or speech output.[24]

Unfortunately, as PD takes its course, the basal ganglia are unable to continue to regulate this function of speech and so voice therapy becomes less effective. In clinicians' experience, more severe PD patients can often still communicate verbally as long as someone else cues them each time they talk to "speak loudly." For those who cannot benefit from this cueing, voice amplification or AAC are alternatives.

Treatment of parkinsonian movement symptoms can come at the cost of increased speech deficits. Long-term effects of using levodopa have led to the use of surgical procedures that may relieve symptoms without associated drug side affects. Pallidotomy for an overactive globus pallidus can reduce tremor and rigidity, but Mourao and colleagues[25] have found that this treatment has little improvement on functional use of communication for PD patients and can actually cause further speech deterioration if the procedure is done bilaterally. Electrical stimulation to an overactive subthalmic nucleus has been shown to improve all the cardinal symptoms of PD.[26] Studies by Pinto and colleagues[27] and Rousseaux and colleagues[28] have demonstrated that although loudness, pitch, and motor movements may improve poststimulation, they do so at the price of decreased intelligibility.

Temporary procedures may provide relief to PD patients without adverse affects. Transoral vocal cord collagen injection for glottal insufficiency may reduce vocal fatigue and be a useful adjunct to voice therapy.[29,30] Dias and colleagues[31] have found evidence that repetitive transcranial stimulation of the primary motor cortex may be beneficial to vocal functioning in PD. Such factors as drug effects, stage of disease, and risk/benefit profile must be taken into consideration when considering treatment options for patients with PD. Among all of the mentioned options, only behavioral therapy has shown a sustained beneficial effect on the voice and speech functions of patients with PD.[32] Voice therapy has been proved the most beneficial to these patients.

Multiple Sclerosis

Hartelius and coworkers,[33] in an analysis of a cohort of 77 patients with multiple sclerosis, found there to be an incidence of dysarthria of 51%, but this depends on the level of severity of the disease overall. The dysarthria results from damage to myelin sheaths in multiple motor and sensory pathways in the central nervous system leading to the bulbar LMNs. Because of its variable pattern of damage, the dysarthria can manifest differently in different patients. It can result from UMN damage, cerebellar damage, or both, with a mixed dysarthria being the most common variety. Not surprisingly, the severity of speech deviation is positively correlated with overall severity of neurologic involvement, type of disease course, and number of years in progression.

The nature of the voice problem also varies. Dysphonia caused by UMN damage tends to be strained, harsh, and loud. Dysphonia caused by ataxia may have adequate vocal quality, but pitch and loudness control are often aberrant. Respiratory support is uneven, contributing to the loudness variability. On sustained phonation, a slow tremor is heard. If the dysarthria has no UMN involvement, muscle tone is low and there is no strained vocal quality. If there is UMN involvement, however, a strained voice quality usually predominates, although it is inconsistent.

Voice therapy is symptomatic. Depending on the voice quality, it may be aimed at relaxation or "ramping" up voice volume and projection. Helping the patient control vocal parameters is the key. Dysarthria caused by multiple sclerosis rarely progresses to the point where the patient is anarthric and needs AAC. Compensatory strategies generally suffice as the dysarthria progresses beyond the point of rehabilitation.

Cerebrovascular Accident or Stroke

Dysphonia from vocal cord paralysis resulting directly from stroke is rare. Most of these cases are associated with brainstem stroke, lateral medullary syndrome, Wallenberg syndrome, and Bernard-Horner syndrome[34] affecting the recurrent laryngeal nerve. Venketasubramanian and colleagues[35] prospectively determined the frequency of vocal cord paresis among first-ever acute ischemic stroke patients. Of the 54 patients with stroke, they found the incidence of vocal cord paralysis to be 20%. Of these, 11.4% of the lacunar infarcts and 16.4% of the cortical and large subcortical groups presented with vocal cord paralysis, affecting the cord contralateral to the side of brain lesion. They also found that 80% of patients with lesions in the lateral medulla suffered from vocal cord paralysis, ipsilateral to the side of the brain lesion.[35] Motor recovery of the paralysis from these etiologies is comparable with motor recovery in general in stroke patients, such that earlier recovery often insinuates a better prognosis.

Whereas brainstem strokes can affect isolated cranial nerves, cerebral hemisphere strokes frequently result in a dysarthria that affects all cranial nerves innervating the speech and voice musculature. A unilateral hemispheric stroke usually results in only minor voice abnormality because of the crossed innervation to the laryngeal region (in contrast to tongue weakness, which is unilaterally weak). A pure cortical stroke also results in a minor dysphonia. In contrast, bilateral strokes (usually multiple strokes) result in a more severe UMN dysarthria that is similar to that of ALS, with slow speech, imprecise articulation, and strained voice quality. Volume is normal or loud and loudness and pitch variability (fine adjustments) are impaired. Respiratory support and control for vocal intensity and stress patterns are reduced. AAC is uncommon in this population because they usually have sufficient speech and voice function to communicate verbally.

Head and Neck Cancer

The ultimate goal of speech rehabilitation after head and neck cancer treatment is functional communication. The goal is to maximize the residual anatomy and physiology to achieve naturalness of the individual's communication. The eventual success depends on the ease with which the patient learns and applies communication strategies, how well their communication is received by family and others, and how satisfied the patient is with the skill.[36] The following section looks at how well two subpopulations of head and neck cancer patients (total glossectomy and total laryngectomy) meet these objectives.

Total glossectomy patients

For relatively small tumors of the tongue and floor of mouth, simple excision with primary closure is often used. This results in a diminution of tongue volume and some tethering of the tongue but relatively good speech. As tumors become more extensive in size with posterior or deep spread, the volume of excision increases and the need for reconstruction beyond primary closure arises. In these cases, larger surgical defects are reconstructed with flaps, grafts, or free tissue transfer. The reconstruction may result in relatively bulky adynamic structures with potential restrictions in tongue mobility and problems with deglutition, speech, and prosthetic rehabilitation.[37]

Other factors that may increase morbidity are mandibular or maxillary resection, radio-therapy, and total laryngectomy.

Vowel and glossal consonant production may be altered by resection of the tongue and the manner of surgical closure.[38–42] The effect on the listener is reduced intelligibility of the speaker's verbal output. Following partial surgery of the tongue with primary closure, intelligibility is least affected, and may be near normal ranging from 70% to 100%. After larger resections that require tongue tip reduction, tethering, or bulky flaps, intelligibility of speech drops markedly to 25% to 40%. Total glossectomy removes the entire tongue and results in intelligibility scores as low as 0% to 8% in some studies.[39,43]

Partial glossectomy may be treated quite successfully with articulation training and prosthodontic palatal appliances.[43,44] Standard speech therapy and prosthetic management are often ineffective for total glossectomy patients because the tongue remnant is small, immobile, or nonexistent and the reconstructed tissue may be adyanmic.[45] Instead, speech therapy is targeted toward teaching compensatory articulatory maneuvers, such as elongating /v/ for /d/ or thrusting the mandible forward for vowels and alternating pause time, phoneme duration, vocal intensity, pitch intonation, and rate of speech.[46] Palatal augmentation prostheses have been found to be less effective for total glossectomy when the reconstructed tongue tissue is adyanmic.[47] Furia and colleagues[39] reported significant improvement in intelligibility for total glossectomy patients after 10 to 16 sessions of compensatory speech therapy. Despite speech therapy and prosthetic augmentation, however, overall intelligibility remained very low ranging from 18% to 42%.[43]

Total glossectomy has earned its reputation as a mutilating surgical procedure because of the associated functional impairments and presumed loss of QOL. Total glossectomy is a radical surgical procedure that impacts significantly on a patient's emotional, physical, and psychosocial state. QOL measurement requires detailed assessment of not only functional outcomes but also their effect on a patient's well-being. QOL studies caution that functional status and QOL are not equivalent, and that function cannot predict QOL.[48]

Although patient functional outcomes are well reported, there has been only one study of QOL in patients having undergone total glossectomy. Ruhl and colleagues[49] reported that highly motivated patients adjust to the functional deficits and have a good QOL after total glossectomy. Maintenance of this QOL was facilitated by the presence of strong emotional support from family and friends in addition to ready access and encouragement from medical and rehabilitation teams. When patients were not well-motivated, lack support, or were not well selected, however, QOL was poor and the functional consequences were overwhelming and devastating.[50]

Some total glossectomy patients may find that they are able successfully to communicate, even with substantially reduced intelligibility. Other patients may not have developed the necessary compensatory skills nor be satisfied with their communication. They commonly report that they are misunderstood when talking with new listeners, when opening up a new topic of conversation, and when talking on the telephone or in noisy environments. Communication may increasingly be reliant on alternate means of communication, such as flip cards, writing, and gestures. A wide range of AAC devices are available for patients who cannot communicate verbally.

Total laryngectomy patients

There are currently three primary options for the voice and speech rehabilitation of laryngectomy patients: (1) esophageal speech, (2) use of an artificial larynx, and (3) TE voice restoration. The choice of communication options for the laryngectomy patient should be made by the individual with input from the physician and speech-language pathologist.

In a large prospective laryngeal preservation study conducted in the Veterans Administration (VA) system, 166 total laryngectomy patients were followed for 2 years posttreatment.[51] Artificial larynx use was found to be the predominant mode of alaryngeal communication across follow-up. Most patients in that study were using an artificial larynx at 1 month post–cancer treatment (85%), and most (55%) were still using it as their primary means of communication as of the last scheduled assessment at 24 months posttreatment. The VA study also found that there was an increase in TE speech acquisition across the 2-year follow-up period, with 2% using secondary TE speech at 1 month post–cancer treatment and 31% using TE speech at 24 months. The noted increase in TE speech use across follow-up seemed to account primarily for the concurrent decrease in artificial larynx use. In studies of TE voice restoration with primary insertion of an indwelling voice prosthesis,[52] the rate of TE usage ranged from 78% to 96% up to 2 years postsurgery. Hillman and colleagues[51] found that no more than 7% of the survivors developed usable esophageal speech at any point in time across the 2-year follow-up period. Only 8% of patients in the VA study were nonvocal at 2 years.

The VA study[51] reported that none of the three modes of alaryngeal speech were judged to be 100% intelligible. TE speech was judged to be 91% intelligible, followed closely by esophageal speech at 90%. Artificial larynx speech was the least intelligible of the modes but still fairly high at 80%.

Ease of use, immediate postlaryngectomy voice production, and elimination of any delay in reacquiring verbal communication have been cited as some reasons for successful artificial larynx use.[53] Failure successfully to use an artificial larynx has been attributed to dissatisfaction with its mechanical sound quality; low volume; reduced intelligibility; inconvenience of using one hand to hold the device; failure to encourage its use; and postsurgery tissue changes or postradiation fibrosis, which preclude the use of the most popular neck-type devices.[53–56]

Success with TE speech has been attributed to the relative ease of the surgical procedure and to the quality of speech, which is fluent, intelligible, and spontaneously acquired with minimal speech therapy.[57,58] Failure to acquire primary or secondary TE speech has been associated with postoperative complications, such as mediastinitis, aspiration pneumonia, persistent pharyngocutaneous fistula, stomal stenosis, salivary aspiration, cellulitis or infection, abscess, cervical spine fracture, false tract creation, pharyngoesophageal stenosis, and pharyngospasm. Behavioral factors, such as difficulty with digital occlusion, gagging, inadvertent prosthesis dislodgment with fistula closure, aspiration of the prosthesis, lack of motivation, and failure to care for the stoma or prosthesis, have also been implicated in the failure to acquire TE speech.[59–64]

Factors that have been associated with successful acquisition of esophageal speech include extent of surgery, positive attitude, psychosocial adjustment, frequency of speech therapy, and family support. Failure to acquire esophageal speech has been associated with lack of motivation, limited physical strength, postoperative radiotherapy, dysphagia, and limited speech therapy.[65,66]

Satisfaction with voice including overall satisfaction with speech quality, telephone use, limitations of interactions, and satisfaction with QOL were reported on by Hillman and coworkers.[51] Results were essentially in line with what might have been predicted based on the findings for speech intelligibility, and also generally in agreement with previous reports dealing with communication satisfaction among alaryngeal speakers. The two groups that displayed the best recovery of intelligibility (ie, TE and esophageal speakers) also showed the best recovery of communication functioning. Artificial larynx users had lower satisfaction than the other two alaryngeal speaker groups. These results are in general agreement with previous research.[67] Satisfaction with nonvocal communication in the VA study was substantially lower than for verbal communication and much more variable over time.

In one study of QOL after total laryngectomy, the presence of a stoma or the use of alaryngeal speech production was not associated with inferior QOL;[68] nor was functional disability correlated with its importance.[69] As part of the VA laryngeal preservation study, Terrell and coworkers[70] reported that the patients who underwent chemotherapy plus radiation reported better QOL scores than the laryngectomies, chiefly because of freedom from pain, better emotional well-being, and lower levels of depression than preservation of voice function.

Cancer of the head and neck often necessitates adjunctive treatments to provide patients with adequate voice use. Tumor debulking can be a useful adjunct to palliate or prepare patients for chemotherapy, radiotherapy, or definite surgery. There are many advantages to the laser as a debulker: rapidity, repeatability, coagulability, atraumaticity, precision, sterilization, and prompt healing. Lim[71] has reported successful debulking in 118 of 120 patients by CO_2 and neodymium:yttrium-aluminum-garnet lasers. Paleri and colleagues[72] reported successful laser debulking in a study of 43 patients, with mean number of debulking per patient to be 1.9, avoiding a tracheotomy in 91%. More recently, Phelan and colleagues[73] have reported successful debulking with the use of microdebriders to re-establish airways in patients with obstructing laryngeal tumors. The avoidance of tracheostomy in these patients is of great benefit because there has been a reported risk of 8% to 41%[74] for tumor seeding of the peristomal wound with resultant recurrence after laryngectomy.

Vocal Cord Paralysis

Vocal fold paralysis may be the presenting symptom of an intrathoracic malignancy. As a result, there may be significant dysfunction of speech, swallowing, respiration, diminished cough reflex with subsequent secretion retention, aspiration, and life-endangering pneumonia. In survey of 42 patients with vocal fold paralysis caused by intrathoracic disease, Bando and colleagues[75] found the most common cause to be lung cancer, followed by thoracic aortic aneurysm, metastatic tumor from other regions, pulmonary and mediastinal tuberculosis, and esophageal cancer. They found that most lesions were easily identified with a chest radiograph, but lesions in the aortopulmonary window were difficult to detect. When in doubt, a contrast-enhanced CT is of great use to detect any mass in this region.

To prevent the sequelae from laryngeal or vagus nerve sectioning during lung cancer resection, Mom and colleagues[76] described a series of 14 patients who underwent concomitant vocal fold medialization during their resection surgery. They were able to achieve an 86% success rate, defined as patients satisfied with the quality of their voice. It may be of great benefit to consider concomitant vocal procedures when thoracic surgery is anticipated to create vocal cord dysfunction.

The most common treatment for vocal fold paralysis is medializing the weak vocal fold toward the midline, for which there are different manners in which this medialization can be achieved. This approach does not address the underlying condition, but rather treats the symptoms. Injection medialization laryngoplasty is one popular option with hyaluronic acid, collagen, and Gelfoam being temporary injectable materials. For more permanent effects, fascia,[77] calcium hydroxyapatite, autologous fat, and more recently titanium[78] can be used for injection. If the paralysis is caused by a terminal disease, only then is Teflon considered because of long-term complications, such as granuloma formation, associated with its use. A type 1 thyroplasty (medialization laryngoplasty) is considered a permanent means to medialize the immobile vocal fold by pushing it medially by external approach. Popular choices for thyroplasty implants include silastic blocks and Gor-Tex. In cases of vocal fold paralysis with a large posterior glottal gap, arytenoid adduction[79] or arytenopexy[80–86] may be indicated in conjunction with type 1 thyroplasty.

Presbyphonia

Voice problems are common in the elderly population. Among retirement community members 65 years of age and older, a prevalence of 20% with 13% having moderate to profound dysphonia was found.[81] In addition, Roy and colleagues[82] demonstrated a lifetime prevalence for a voice disorder in 47% of elderly 65 years of age and older. Dysphonia was often chronic with 60% of the 29.1% with a current voice disorder having the problem for more than 4 weeks. Voice problems have a significant impact on elderly patients' QOL. Over a 5-year span among 50 to 81 year olds, altered acoustic properties of the voice, increased vocal roughness, increased patient-reported vocal instability, and avoidance of social events was noted.[83] Hence, appropriate diagnosis and treatment is necessary.

Presbyphonia refers to voice changes related to aging of the larynx. Patients with presbyphonia may complain of a weak voice, change in pitch, decreased projection, vocal fatigue, the sense of taking more effort to speak, and altered quality of the voice. These alterations are related to a multitude of changes affecting the phonatory system. The larynx descends in the neck, and the laryngeal cartilages ossify, altering the resonant properties of the larynx and pharynx.[84,85] Decreased muscle bulk with fatty degeneration and altered distribution of muscle fiber type has been shown.[86,87] Alterations within the lamina propria and connective tissue of the vocal fold affect the vibratory characteristics and in conjunction with muscle atrophy produce a bowed membranous vocal fold with possible glottal insufficiency during phonation.[84] Secretions, which provide important lubrication during vocal fold vibration, decrease and become thicker.[88] Lastly, one's overall health seems related to vocal function.[89]

Although presbyphonia is an important cause of dysphonia, other etiologies must also be considered in the elderly population. The prevalence of presbyphonia among the elderly ranges from 4%[90] to 30%.[91] Woo and colleagues[90] have noted that certain diseases are more common among the elderly with a higher prevalence of neurologic voice disorders and less functional voice disorders in patients older than 60 years. In addition, multiple factors, such as vocal hygiene, decreased respiratory support, medication effects, and other medical problems, may cause dysphonia.[90] Hence, a thorough evaluation is essential to diagnose and treat accurately elderly patients presenting with dysphonia.

Treatment for presbyphonia includes both voice therapy and surgical options. Because of the voice changes associated with aging, patients may develop compensatory strategies, such as straining, which may worsen the dysphonia. Although voice therapy aimed at reducing the compensatory behaviors may unmask the glottal incompetence caused by the atrophic vocal folds,[84] voice therapy has been shown to improve voice-related QOL in patients 60 years of age and older.[92] A total of 74% of patients improved with voice therapy, 21% were worse after voice therapy, and 5% reported no change from voice therapy.[92] The influence of the degree of glottal insufficiency on voice therapy outcomes and the ability to preselect which patients will benefit from voice therapy requires further investigation. Furthermore, voice therapy aimed at strengthening, such as Lee Silverman Voice Treatment, may be an effective treatment for presbyphonia. Although three patients with presbyphonia demonstrated improved loudness following Lee Silverman Voice Treatment, more study is necessary.[93] Despite the limitations, voice therapy is a valid, noninvasive, first-line treatment for elderly patients with dysphonia.

When voice therapy does not improve the voice, surgical options should be entertained. To address the glottal insufficiency, bilateral medialization laryngoplasty procedures have been developed. A multitude of injection materials are available for injection laryngoplasty.[94] Collagen injection bilaterally has resulted in improved voice perceptually and improved voice handicap as measured on the Voice Handicap Index.[95] Additionally, bilateral medialization laryngoplasty with silastic implants is also a viable option. Patients with presbyphonia had improved voice based on self-report and clinician ratings.[96] Certain changes in implant design must be taken into consideration in treating vocal fold atrophy compared with vocal fold paralysis. Avoiding overcorrection anteriorly and reducing the posterior flange and shortening the anteroposterior dimension are important adjustments for presbyphonic patients.[96] Too large a posterior flange could impinge on the arytenoid, decreasing its mobility. Gor-Tex has also been a useful material for bilateral medialization laryngoplasty procedures.[97]

Despite the versatility of bilateral medialization laryngoplasty, simply correcting the glottal insufficiency may not fully correct the voice problem. Such procedures mainly address the glottal gap in the axial plane. Yet, because of the atrophic changes of the vocal fold muscle and lamina propria, volume loss also occurs in the coronal plane.[84] Simply repositioning atrophic vocal folds does not address the volume loss to the vocal folds. A combination of procedures, such as bilateral medialization laryngoplasty with implants and injection to restore bulk, may be required. Postma and colleagues[98,99] noted that 35% of patients required lipoinjections after bilateral silastic medialization laryngoplasty to optimize the outcome. Furthermore, such advances as using growth factors and muscle stem cell injections into atrophic vocal folds may prove to be exciting potential future interventions.

REFERENCES

1. Ruotsalainen JH, Sellman J, Lehto L, et al. Interventions for preventing voice disorders in adults. Cochrane Database Syst Rev 2007;(4):CD006372, Review.
2. Happ MB, Roesch T, Kagan SH. Communication needs, methods, and perceived voice quality following head and neck surgery: a literature review. Cancer Nurs 2004;27(1):1–9, Review.
3. Kantner CE, West R. Phonetics. New York: Harper and Brothers; 1941.
4. Esposito, S.J. Speech and palatolpharyngeal function. In: Zlotolow, I, Esposito S.J, Beumer J, editors. Proceedings of the first international congress on maxillofacial prosthetics. June 1, 1995; New York: Memorial Sloan-Kettering Cancer Center; 1995. p. 43–8.
5. Ramig LO, Sapir S, Countryman S, et al. Intensive voice treatment (LSVT) for patients with Parkinson's disease: a 2 year follow up. J Neurol Neurosurg Psychiatr 2001;71(4):493–8.
6. Joseph C Stemple, Leslie E Glaze, Klaben Bernice Gerdeman. Clinical voice pathology: theory and management. Singular Press, Thomson Learning, San Diego(CA), 2000.
7. Roy N. Functional dysphonia. Curr Opin Otolaryngol Head Neck Surg 2003;11(3): 144–8, Review.
8. Aronson AE. Extrinsic muscular tension in patients with voice disorders. J Voice 2004;18(2):275.

9. Verdolini K, Druker DG, Palmer PM, et al. Laryngeal adduction in resonant voice. J Voice 1998;12(3):315–27.
10. Stemple JC, Lee L, D'Amico B, et al. Efficacy of vocal function exercises as a method of improving voice production. J Voice 1994;8(3):271–8.
11. Ball L, Beukelman D, Bilyeu D, et al. Duration of AAC technology use by persons with ALS. Journal of Medical Speech Language Pathology, in press.
12. Beukelman DR, Ball LJ. Improving AAC use for persons with acquired neurogenic disorders: understanding human and engineering factors. Assist Technol 2002; 14:33–44.
13. Beukelman DR, Fager S, Ball L, et al. AAC for adults with acquired neurological conditions: a review. Augment Altern Commun 2007;23(3):230–42.
14. Scott A, McPhee M. Speech and language therapy. In: Oliver D, Borasio GD, Walsh D, editors. Palliative care in amyotrophic lateral sclerosis: from diagnosis to bereavement. 2nd edition. Oxford: Oxford University Press; 2006. p. 213–27.
15. Kubler A, Nijboer F, Mellinger J, et al. Patients with ALS can use sensorimotor rhythms to operate a brain-computer interface. Neurology 2005;64:1775–7.
16. Esposito SJ, Mitsumoto H, Shanks M. Use of palatal lift and palatal augmentation prostheses to improve dysarthria in patients with amyotrophic lateral sclerosis: a case series. J Prosthet Dent 2000;83(1):90–8.
17. Hartelius L, Svensson P. Speech and swallowing symptoms associated with Parkinson's disease and multiple sclerosis a survey. Folia Phoniatr Logop 1994; 46:9–17.
18. de Angelis EC, Mourao LF, Ferraz HB, et al. Effect of voice rehabilitation on oral communication of Parkinson's disease patients. Acta Neurol Scand 1997;96(4): 199–205.
19. Blonsky ER, Logeman JA, Boshes B, et al. Comparison of speech and swallowing function in patients with tremor disorders and in normal geriatric patients: a cinefluorographic study. J Gerontol 1975;30:299–303.
20. Perez KS, Ramig LO, Smith ME, et al. The Parkinson's larynx tremor and videostroboscopic findings. J Voice 1996;10:354–61.
21. Trail M, Fox C, Ramig LO, et al. Speech treatment for Parkinson's disease. NeuroRehabilitation 2005;20(3):205–21.
22. Schumacher J, Rosenbek J. Behavioral treatment of hypokinetic dysarthria: further investigation of aided speech. ASHA 1986;28:145.
23. Steinfeld E. Architecture as a communication medium. In: Lubinski R, Higginbotham DJ, editors. Communication technologies for the elderly: vision, hearing, and speech. San Diego: Singular Publishing Group; 1997. p. 262–94.
24. Beukelman DR, Yorkston KM, Reichle J. Augmentative and alternative communication for adults with acquired neurologic disorders. Baltimore: Paul H. Brooks Publishing Co; 2000. p. 257–60.
25. Mourao LF, Aguiar PM, Ferraz FA, et al. Acoustic voice assessment in Parkinson's disease patients submitted to posteroventral pallidotomy. Arq Neuropsiquiatr 2005;63(1):20–5.
26. Volkmann J, Sturm V, Weiss P, et al. Bilateral high-frequency stimulation of the internal globus pallidus in advanced Parkinson's disease. Ann Neurol 1998;44: 953–61.
27. Pinto S, Ozsancak C, Tripoliti E, et al. Treatments for dysarthria in Parkinson's disease. Lancet Neurol 2004;3(9):547–56.
28. Rousseaux M, Krystkowiak P, Kozlowski O, et al. Effects of subthalamic nucleus stimulation on parkinsonian dysarthria and speech intelligibility. J Neurol 2004; 251(3):327–34.

29. Sewall GK, Jiang J, Ford CN. Clinical evaluation of Parkinson's-related dysphonia. Laryngoscope 2006;116(10):1740–4.
30. Berke GS, Gerratt B, Kreiman J, et al. Treatment of Parkinson hypophonia with percutaneous collagen augmentation. Laryngoscope 1999;109(8):1295–9.
31. Dias AE, Barbosa ER, Coracini K, et al. Effects of repetitive transcranial magnetic stimulation on voice and speech in Parkinson's disease. Acta Neurol Scand 2006; 113(2):92–9.
32. Merati AL, Heman-Ackah YD, Abaza M. Common movement disorders affecting the larynx: a report from the Neurolaryngology Committee of the AAO-HNS. Otolaryngol Head Neck Surg 2005;133(5):654–65.
33. Hartelius L, Runmarker B, Andersen O. Prevalence and characteristics of dysarthria in a multiple-sclerosis incidence cohort: relation to neurological data. Folia Phoniatr Logop 2000;52(4):160–77.
34. Rigueiro-Veloso MT, Pego-Reigosa R, Branas-Fernandez F, et al. Wallenberg syndrome: a review of 25 cases. Rev Neurol 1997;25(146):1561–4.
35. Venketasubramanian N, Seshadri R, Chee N. Vocal cord paresis in acute ischemic stroke. Cerebrovasc Dis 1999;9(3):157–62.
36. Carpenter M. Treatment decisions in alaryngeal speech. In: Salmon S, editor. Alaryngeal speech rehabilitation: for clinicians by clinicians. 2nd edition. Austin: PRO-ED; 1999. p. 55–77.
37. Silverman S. Oral cancer. 4th edition. Hamilton: Decker; 1998.
38. Skelly M, Donaldson R, Fust R. Glossectomee speech rehabilitation. Springfield: Thomas; 1973.
39. Furia C, Kowalski L, Latorre M, et al. Speech intelligibility after glossectomy and speech rehabilitation. Arch Otolaryngol Head Neck Surg 2001;127:877–83.
40. Messengill R, Maxwell S, Pickrell K. An analysis of articulation following partial and total glossectomy. J Speech Hear Disord 1970;35:170–3.
41. Pauloski B, Logemann J, Colangelo L, et al. Surgical variables affecting speech in treated patients with oral and oropharyngeal cancer. Laryngoscope 1998; 108(6):908–16.
42. Savariaux C, Perrier P, Pape D, et al. Speech production after glossectomy and reconstructive lingual surgery: a longitudinal study. In: Proceedings of the 2nd international workshop on models and analysis of vocal emissions for biomedical applications (MAVEBA). Firenze: 2001.
43. Gillis R, Leonard R. Prosthetic treatment for speech and swallowing in patients with total glossectomy. J Prosthet Dent 1983;50:808–14.
44. Robbins K, Bowman J, Jacob R. Postglossectomy deglutitory and articulatory rehabilitation with palatal augmentation prosthesis. Arch Otolaryngol Head Neck Surg 1987;113:1214–8.
45. Skelly M, Donaldson R, Fust R, et al. Changes in phonatory aspects of glossectomee intelligibility through vocal parameter manipulation. J Speech Hear Disord 1972;37:379–89.
46. Skelly M, Spector D, Donaldson R, et al. Compensatory physiologic phonetics for the glossectomee. J Speech Hear Disord 1971;36:101–12.
47. Leonard R, Gillis R. Differential effects of speech prostheses in glossectomy patients. J Prosthet Dent 1990;64:701–8.
48. Cella D. Quality of life: concepts and definition. J Pain Symptom Manage 1994;9:186–92.
49. Ruhl C, Gleich L, Gluckman J. Survival, function, and quality of life after total glossectomy. Laryngoscope 1997;107(10):1316–21.
50. Bova R, Cheung I, Coman W. Total glossectomy: is it justified? ANZ J Surg 2004; 74(3):134–8.

51. Hillman R, Walsh M, Wolf G, et al. Functional outcomes following treatment for advanced laryngeal cancer. Part I—Voice preservation in advanced laryngeal cancer; Part II—Laryngectomy rehabilitation: the state of the art in the VA System. Ann Otol Rhinol Laryngol 1998;72(Suppl):1–27.
52. Chone C, Gripp F, Spina A, et al. Primary versus secondary tracheoesophageal puncture for speech rehabilitation in total laryngectomy: long-term results with indwelling voice prosthesis. Otolaryngol Head Neck Surg 2005;133:89–93.
53. Bennett S, Weinberg B. Acceptability ratings of normal, esophageal, and artificial larynx speech. J Speech Hear Res 1973;16:608–15.
54. Merwin G, Goldstein L, Rothman H. A comparison of speech using artificial larynx and tracheoesophageal puncture with valve in the same speaker. Laryngoscope 1985;95:730–4.
55. Verdolini K, Skinner M, Patton T, et al. Effect of amplification on the intelligibility of speech produced with an electrolarynx. Laryngoscope 1985;95:720–6.
56. Weiss M, Yeni-Komshian G, Heinz J. Acoustical and perceptual characteristics of speech produced with an electronic artificial larynx. J Acoust Soc Am 1979;65(5):1298–308.
57. Blom E, Singer M, Hamaker R. A prospective study of tracheoesophageal speech. Arch Otolaryngol Head Neck Surg 1986;112:440–7.
58. Doyle P. Foundations of voice and speech rehabilitation following laryngectomy. San Diego: Singular; 1994.
59. Andrews C, Mickel R, Hanson D, et al. Major complications following tracheoesophageal puncture for voice rehabilitation. Laryngoscope 1987;97:562–7.
60. Blom E, Pauloski B, Hamaker R. Functional outcome after surgery for prevention of pharyngospasms in tracheoesophageal speakers: Part I. Speech characteristics. Laryngoscope 1995;105:1093–103.
61. Izdebski K, Reed C, Ross J, et al. Problems with tracheoesophageal fistula voice restoration in totally laryngectomized patients: a review of 95 cases. Arch Otolaryngol Head Neck Surg 1994;120:840–5.
62. Maniglia A, Lundy D, Casiano R, et al. Speech restoration and complications of primary versus secondary tracheoesophageal puncture following total laryngectomy. Laryngoscope 1989;99:489–91.
63. McConnel F, Duck S. Indications for tracheoesophageal puncture speech rehabilitation. Laryngoscope 1986;96:1065–8.
64. Quer M, Burgues-Vila J, Garcia-Crespillo P. Primary tracheoesophageal puncture vs. esophageal speech. Arch Otolaryngol Head Neck Surg 1992;118:188–90.
65. Gates G, Ryan W, Cantu E, et al. Current status of laryngectomee rehabilitation: II. Causes of failure. Am J Otol 1982;3(1):8–14.
66. Richardson J. Surgical and radiological effects upon the development of speech after total laryngectomy. Ann Otol Rhinol Laryngol 1981;90(3 Pt 1):294–7.
67. Clements K, Rassekh C, Seikaly H, et al. Communication after laryngectomy: an assessment of patient satisfaction. Arch Otolaryngol Head Neck Surg 1997;123:493–6.
68. Harranz J, Gavilan J. Psychosocial adjustment after laryngeal cancer surgery. Ann Otol Rhinol Laryngol 1999;108(10):990–7.
69. Deleyiannis F, Weymuller E, Coltrera M, et al. Quality of life after laryngectomy: are functional disabilities important? Head Neck 1999;21:319–24.
70. Terrell J, Fisher S, Wolf G. Long-term quality of life after treatment of laryngeal cancer. Arch Otolaryngol Head Neck Surg 1998;124:964–71.
71. Lim RY. Laser tumor debulking. W V Med J 1989;85(12):530–2.
72. Paleri V, Stafford FW, Sammut MS. Laser debulking in malignant upper airway obstruction. Head Neck 2005;27(4):296–301.

73. Phelan E, Lang E, Mahesh BN, et al. Powered instrumentation in obstructing laryngeal tumors. J Laryngol Otol 2007;121(3):293–5.
74. Halfpenny W, McGurk M. Stomal recurrence following temporary tracheostomy. J Laryngol Otol 2001;115:202–4.
75. Bando H, Nishio T, Bamba H, et al. Vocal fold paralysis as a sign of chest diseases: a 15-year retrospective study. World J Surg 2006;30(3):293–8.
76. Mom T, Filaire M, Advenier D, et al. Concomitant type I thyroplasty and thoracic operations for lung cancer: preventing respiratory complications associated with vagus or recurrent laryngeal nerve injury. J Thorac Cardiovasc Surg 2001;121(4):642–8.
77. Nishiyama K, Hirose H, Nagai H, et al. Endoscopic vocal cord medialization: a new surgical technique without neck incision for laryngeal palsy. Acta Otolaryngol 2005;125(10):1134–6.
78. Schneider B, Denk DM, Bigenzahn W. Functional results after external vocal fold medialization thyroplasty with the titanium vocal fold medialization implant. Laryngoscope 2003;113(4):628–34.
79. Isshiki N, Tanabe M, Sawadw M. Arytenoid adduction for unilateral vocal cord paralysis. Arch Otolaryngol 1978;104:555–8.
80. Zeitels SM, Hillman RE, Desloge RB. Cricothyroid subluxation: a new innovation for enhancing the voice with laryngoplastic phonosurgery. Ann Otol Rhinol Laryngol 1999;108(12):1126–31.
81. Golub JS, Chen PH, Otto KJ, et al. Prevalence of perceived dysphonia in a geriatric population. J Am Geriatr Soc 2006;54:1736–9.
82. Roy N, Stemple J, Merrill RM, et al. Epidemiology of voice disorders in the elderly: preliminary findings. Laryngoscope 2007;117:628–33.
83. Verdonck-de Leeuw IM, Mahieu HF. Vocal aging and the impact on daily life: a longitudinal study. J Voice 2004;193–202.
84. Woodson GE. The aging larynx. In: Ossoff RH, Shapshay SM, Woodson GE, et al, editors. The larynx. 1st edition. Philadelphia (PA): Lippincott Williams & Wilkins; 2003. p. 251–6.
85. Linville WE, Fisher GB. Acoustic characteristics of women's voices with advanced age. J Gerontol 1985;40:324–30.
86. Kahane JC. Connective tissue changes and their effects on voice. J Voice 1987;1:27–30.
87. Malmgren LT, Fisher PJ, Bookman LM, et al. Age-related changes in muscle fiver types in the human thyroarytenoid muscle: an immunohistochemical and stereological study using confocal laser scanning microscopy. Otolaryngol Head Neck Surg 1999;121:441–51.
88. Sato K, Hirano M. Age-related changes in the human laryngeal glands. Ann Otol Rhinol Laryngol 1998;197:525–9.
89. Ramig LO, Ringel R. Effects of physiological aging on selected acoustic characteristics of voice. J Speech Lang Hear Res 1983;26:22–30.
90. Woo P, Casper J, Colton R, et al. Dysphonia in the aging: physiology versus disease. Laryngoscope 1992;102:139–44.
91. Hagen P, Lyons GD, Nuss DW. Dysphonia in the elderly: diagnosis and management of age-related voice changes. Southampt Med J 1996;89:204–7.
92. Berg EE, Hapner E, Klein A, et al. Voice therapy improves quality of life in age-related dysphonia: a case-control study. J Voice 2008;22:70–4.
93. Ramig LO, Gray S, Baker K, et al. The aging voice: a review, treatment data, and familial and genetic perspectives. Folia Phoniatr Logop 2001;53:252–65.

94. King JM, Simpson CB. Modern injection augmentation for glottic insufficiency. Curr Opin Otolaryngol Head Neck Surg 2007;15:153–8.
95. Remacle M, Lawson G. Results with collagen injection into the vocal folds for medialization. Curr Opin Otolaryngol Head Neck Surg 2007;15:148–52.
96. Postma GN, Blalock PD, Koufman JA. Bilateral medialization laryngoplasty. Laryngoscope 1998;108:1429–34.
97. Zeitels SM, Mauri M, Dailey SH. Medialization laryngoplasty with Gore-Tex for voice restoration secondary to glottal incompetence: indication and observation. Ann Otol Rhinol Laryngol 2003;112:180–4.
98. Hirano S, Bless DM, del Rio AM, et al. Therapeutic potential of growth factors for aging voice. Laryngoscope 2004;114:2161–7.
99. Halum SL, Naidu M, Delo DM, et al. Injection of autologous muscle stem cells (myoblasts) for the treatment of vocal fold paralysis: a pilot study. Laryngoscope 2007;117:917–22.

Anosmia: Loss of Smell in the Elderly

Denis Lafreniere, MD, FACS[a],*, Norman Mann, MD[b,c]

KEYWORDS

• Smell loss • Anosmia • Aging

At least 35 million people aged 65 years or older are living in the United States, accounting for 13% of the US population. This number is estimated to increase to 75 million by 2030.[1] Although not a life-threatening problem, the loss of taste and smell can result in significant changes in appetite and food preferences and, in turn, affect the quality of life and nutritional status in the elderly population.[2,3] Intact smell is an important warning system that alerts us to the presence of leaking gas, smoke, food spoilage, and pollution. The absolute sensitivity to odor and the appreciation of suprathreshold odors decline with increasing age.[4] In many elderly patients there is unawareness of actual smell loss. Nardin and colleagues[5] showed that 77% of older patients with smell loss reported normal smell sensitivity. Smell sensation deficits occur in many neurodegenerative diseases such as Alzheimer's and Parkinson's disease which typically affect the elderly.[6] The etiology of smell loss in older patients has yet to be completely defined. The loss of smell sensitivity can be due to conditions that could affect any step in the olfactory process from the transport of odors up to the olfactory cleft to the central processing of olfactory information.

ANATOMY AND PHYSIOLOGY OF THE SENSE OF SMELL

Odors reach the olfactory epithelium orthonasally via the nose or retronasally via the oropharnx. Retronasal function is essential for the proper appreciation of flavor of food. Odorants are detected when they bind to receptor proteins present in the olfactory receptor neurons which are located in the olfactory epithelium in the dorsal aspect of the nasal cavity (**Fig. 1**). These receptor cells have nonmotile ciliary projections that express one of several hundred different olfactory receptor proteins.[7] The olfactory receptor function is dependent on the composition of the mucous layer that is produced by the Bowman's glands and sustentacular cells. This mucous layer

[a] Division of Otolaryngology, Department of Surgery, University of Connecticut Health Center, 263 Farmington Avenue, MC-6228, Farmington, CT 06030-6228, USA
[b] Department of Medicine, University of Connecticut Health Center, 263 Farmington Avenue, MC-1718, Farmington, CT 06030-1718, USA
[c] Taste and Smell Clinic, University of Connecticut Health Center, 263 Farmington Avenue, Farmington, CT 06030, USA
* Corresponding author.
E-mail address: lafreniere@nso.uchc.edu (D. Lafreniere).

Otolaryngol Clin N Am 42 (2009) 123–131
doi:10.1016/j.otc.2008.09.001
0030-6665/08/$ – see front matter © 2009 Elsevier Inc. All rights reserved.

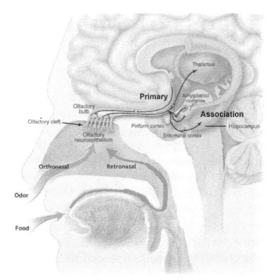

Fig.1. Anatomy of olfaction. Odors reach the olfactory cleft via the orthonasal or retronasal route. Odors bind to receptor proteins on the olfactory receptor neurons in the olfactory epithelium, which depolarizes the cell and sends the signal to the olfactory bulb. In the bulb the neuron synapses and propagates the signal centrally to primary and associational regions where the information is integrated with other sensory information. (*From* Davenport RJ. The flavor of aging. Sci Aging Knowl Environ 2004;12:ns1. [DOI: 10.1126/sageke.2004.12.ns1]. Illustration: K. Sutliff. Modified with permission from AAAS, www.sciencemag.org.)

contains mucopolysaccharides, enzymes, and immune factors which can help modify olfactory stimulants but also have a role in the detoxification of inhaled substances, the protection of other organs, and the activation of toxicants.[8] The composition of nasal secretions can change dramatically with inflammation, toxic exposure, or disease. Because the ciliary projections of the olfactory receptor neurons are nonmotile, mucociliary clearance of the olfactory cleft is solely dependent on the ciliary function of the respiratory epithelium. Normal respiratory ciliary function can be reduced by toxic exposures such as cigarette smoke.[8]

Activation of an olfactory receptor neuron results in G-protein CAMP cascade, which leads to cell depolarization. Olfactory receptor neurons expressing the same receptor proteins converge onto the same loci in the olfactory bulb. This process ensures transfer of a given odorant signal to a specific set of mitral cells in the olfactory bulb.[7] The signal can then propagate centrally via the olfactory tracts and the lateral olfactory striae and terminate in the amygdala and the primary olfactory cortex of the uncus. Projections can then connect to the association olfactory cortex of the parahippocampal gyrus and the entorhinal. The parahippocampal gyrus receives fibers from the cingulate gyrus via the cingulum and projects into the hippocampus.[9] These primary and associative areas are referred to as the pyriform cortex (see **Fig. 1**). The amygdala receives connections from the middle and inferior temporal gyri important for semantic processing. Damage to the pyriform cortex could impair smell at the perceptual or sensory level. Damage to the temporal cortical-amygdala connections could impair associative capabilities.

Mammalian olfactory epithelium maintains the ability to replace olfactory neurons lost via injury.[10] Olfactory neurogenesis, stimulated by the death of olfactory receptor neurons, begins with the maturation of progenitor cells. These precursor cells mature and extend axons through the cribriform plate which synapse within the olfactory bulb where they derive trophic factors needed for long-term survival.[10] Olfactory receptor cells are bipolar neurons directly exposed to the external environment and the dangers of that environment, including injury from infection, inflammatory, and noxious chemical agents. This environmental exposure results in a regular turnover of olfactory receptor cells. Cell death frequently occurs via the process of apoptosis. Apoptosis is a programmed active process that usually begins with the receipt of a death signal that then activates intrinsic enzymes which ultimately lead to cell death. This mechanism is used for the removal of aged or damaged cells, immune regulation, and cancer surveillance and in response to injury. Recent studies by Kern and colleagues[11] have demonstrated increases in levels of capsase 3, the dominant executioner enzyme in the apoptotic pathway, in the olfactory epithelial cells of patients with nasal sinus disease as well as in mice models of traumatic smell loss. This finding suggests an increase in programmed cell death in these conditions.

SMELL LOSS WITH AGING

Many studies have shown a decrease in olfactory ability in humans with advancing age.[12–18] Researchers have documented this loss using several different psychophysical measures, including odor detection (threshold), quality discrimination, and odor identification. The detection of suprathreshold odors also appears to decrease with age.[4] These decreases in olfactory ability are noted in both sexes after the age of 69 years; however, women are better at identifying odors than men at all ages. After the age of 80 years, 62% to 80% of subjects tested showed major olfactory impairment, with 50% of subjects completely anosmic.[4,19,20]

Mucous Layer

The ability to perceive odors may be modified by changes in the mucous layer in the olfactory cleft that occurs with increasing age. The mucous layer influences odor deposition and clearance rates. Studies have shown a decline in hydration and secretion of mucus in the elderly population.[21]

Modification of the olfactory xenobiotic metabolism may have a role in the decline of smell sensitivity over the years that the mucosa is exposed to the environment. Many common environmental exposures may alter nasal enzymatic activity, which could enhance individual variations in responses to toxic exposures.[8] These alterations can be due to direct exposure to chemicals that induce or inhibit nasal enzymes or from toxic insults that may alter the olfactory mucosa. Exposure to heavy metals such as manganese can lead to smell loss that can occur at a subtle degree, often leaving the patient unaware of any impairment, similar to the symptoms seen in patients with Alzheimer's and Parkinson's disease.[22,23] Toxic exposures over a lifetime could have a role in age-related smell loss. Cigarette smoke is another pollutant that can alter olfaction. Rhondase, an enzyme responsible for cyanide metabolism, shows a 50% reduction in activity in smokers when compared with nonsmokers.[8] Some odorous stimuli are potentially harmful to the olfactory mucosa if they reach high enough concentrations and remain in the olfactory cleft for prolonged periods of time. Volatile substances with potentially harmful effects usually are presented to the olfactory epithelium for short periods and in low enough concentrations to avoid causing harm; however, the reduced mucociliary movement, reduced hydration, thinner epithelium, and decreased enzymatic activity seen in older olfactory epithelium may allow these substances to contribute to epithelial damage.[7]

Changes in Olfactory Epithelium

Histologic studies show a replacement of olfactory epithelium with respiratory epithelium during aging (**Fig. 2**).[24] Animal studies have shown a thinning of the olfactory mucosa with age, a decrease in the number of olfactory neurons present, and an increase in the irregularity of the respiratory/olfactory mucosal border.[25] It appears there may be an increase in natural cell turnover via the apoptotic pathway in older mice. Robinson and colleagues[10] reported increased expression of the procapsase 3 gene in older rats. This gene leads to production of capsase 3, the major executioner enzyme in the apoptotic pathway. This gene also appears to be up-regulated in bulbectomized mice, which would contribute to cell death in traumatic anosmia. An increase in apoptosis, suggested by increased levels of capsase 3, is also noted in rats exposed to cigarette smoke when compared with normal controls.[26] This increase in the executioner enzyme was noted in the epithelium and nerve bundles in the lamina propria, showing an increase in apoptosis in the cell bodies and axon bundles of mature olfactory sensory neurons. The increase in capsase 3 was also noted in the progenitor basal cells and the supporting cells of the exposed epithelium, which would impact the neurogenesis of replacement sensory neurons.

The question remains to what degree the histologic changes seen in the aging olfactory mucosa are due to years of environmental exposure versus other changes in the intrinsic controls of neurogenesis. Rawson and colleagues[27] found that it was just as likely to obtain functional olfactory neurons from the olfactory mucosa of older patients as from younger patients, suggesting that if there is a loss of olfactory neurons in older subjects it is distributed equally throughout the mucosa. Other studies such as that by Loo and colleagues[28] suggest that exposure to the airflow environment may have a role along with changes in neurogenesis seen with aging. In these studies, Loo and colleagues[28] noted a difference in the histologic appearance of the anterior olfactory cells when compared with the middle and posterior cells in aged rats. In older hybrid rats protected from external pollutants, the number of mature olfactory neurons did not change markedly as a function of age in the middle and posterior aspects of the mucosa. The distribution of basal cells in this area was similar to that in younger

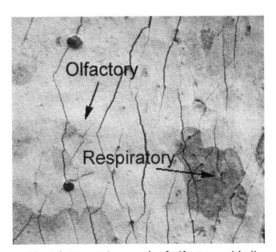

Fig. 2. Low-power scanning electron micrograph of olfactory epithelium. Lighter areas are olfactory neuroepithelium. Dark patches are areas of respiratory epithelium. Patches of respiratory epithelium are more numerous in older subjects.

rats; however, the number of immature olfactory neurons was fewer in the middle and posterior zones of the older animals when compared with the younger rats. The results demonstrate a decrease in the population of immature neurons relative to the population of mature neurons. This finding is in contrast to the anterior-dorsal septal cells, which had a higher density of proliferating basal cells than seen in younger rats. The epithelium in the anterior dorsal aspect was abnormal in several respects, with some areas grossly distorted. The number of immature neurons increased and the number of mature neurons decreased as a function of age. The decrease in proliferating cells in the posterior aspect of the epithelium in aging rats suggests some intrinsic controls on neurogenesis may be unrelated to the rate of neuronal death. The anterior epithelium in older rats showed damaged mucosa with a decrease in mature neurons, disordered mucosa, and an increase in immature neurons. This finding suggests that, in these environmentally protected rats, there may be a role for airflow alone contributing to the changes, because similar findings are noted on the open side of rats with unilateral nares occlusion.[28]

Central Connections

Intact sensation of olfactory stimuli relies not only on intact olfactory receptor neurons but on intact and appropriate synapses as the signal moves centrally. Christensen and colleagues[29] have shown that nerve transection disrupts normal targeting of the olfactory bulb by the immature neuronal cell. Other factors that contribute to peripheral neuron deterioration, such as smoking and viruses, may also ultimately have a role in the development of aberrant synapses and may contribute to the loss of olfactory bulb mitral cells with age. In the olfactory bulb, the number of mitral cells continuously decreases with age. It is estimated that the adult olfactory bulb contains about 60,000 mitral cells at age 25 years and only 14,500 at age 95 years.[30]

Neurodegenerative Disorders

Damage to the cells of the olfactory bulb and central pathways is seen in many neurodegenerative diseases that affect the elderly. Smell sensation deficits occur in many neurodegenerative diseases, such as Alzheimer's disease, Parkinson's disease, multiple system atrophy, Huntington's disease, multiple sclerosis, and amyotrophic lateral sclerosis.[6,9,31–33] The incidence and degree of smell loss in these patients can be variable and often is dependent on disease severity. The characteristics of the smell deficit are dependent on the site of the lesion.

Alzheimer's disease is the most common neurodegenerative disorder in humans and is the major cause of dementia in the elderly.[6] The olfactory deficits seen in these patients are usually perceptual. Neurofibrillary tangles composed of an abnormally phosphorylated fibrillar microtubule-associated protein (tau) have been implicated as one of the pathologic lesions in the brain tissue of patients with Alzheimer's disease. The Braak stage has been used to describe the severity of this pathology, with stages 5 and 6 being the most severe.[34] Several studies have demonstrated similar tau pathology in the olfactory bulbs of patients with definitive Alzheimer's disease. This tau pathology is seen early in the disease process and increases with the severity of the disease.[31,33] Clinical dementia is highly correlated with both Braak stage and olfactory system tau scores. Attems and colleagues[31] have suggested that in the future biopsies of the olfactory mucosa looking for tau pathology may be useful in determining the risk of future cognitive decline. Early stage Alzheimer's disease can result in a loss of odor detection and odor discrimination as the tau pathology has more of a peripheral effect that is separate from any cognitive decline. Olfactory loss in these patients can be seen as an early feature of the disease.[9] As the disease progresses and more tau pathology is seen in the central olfactory areas, patients ultimately develop odor identification deficits. Individuals who are heterozygous or homozygous for the apolipoprotein E (APOE 4) genotype have a higher risk of developing Alzheimer's disease.[33] Tsuboi and colleagues[33] showed a correlation between APOE 4 and tau pathology in the olfactory bulb in a gene dose-dependent manner. Nondemented carriers of APOE 4 have worse olfactory identification scores than APOE 4–negative persons. Olfactory dysfunction and APOE 4 are associated with a greater risk of cognitive decline.

Parkinson's disease is the second most common neurodegenerative disease in humans. Olfactory dysfunction is a significant feature of Parkinson's disease, and testing of smell identification can be useful in differentiating Parkinson's disease from other extrapyramidal disorders such as progressive supranuclear palsy in which odor identification and threshold remain intact. Olfactory abnormalities are detected early in Parkinson's disease but remain stable as the disease progresses.[33] Lewy bodies are the pathologic lesions seen. They are composed of aggregated fibrillar alpha synuclein and are seen in the olfactory bulb and the lower brain stem. Lewy bodies then develop in the midbrain, limbic system, and neocortex.[32] Olfactory dysfunction is similar in different types of Parkinson's disease.[35] Problems with odor recognition have been noted in patients. Masoka and colleagues[32] noted that patients who had Parkinson's disease needed a higher odor concentration to recognize an odor. Semantic processing is also lower than normal in these patients.[32]

Other neurodegenerative disorders such as semantic dementia and frontotemporal dementia which have no olfactory nerve or pyriform cortex pathology can show normal odor perception and discrimination but impaired odor identification. This characteristic can point to the central pathology of the temporal lobes seen in semantic dementia, which have a role in olfactory memory, and that of the frontal lobes seen in frontotemporal dementia, which are involved in odor processing.[9] The orbitofrontal areas are implicated in the determination of pleasantness of odors and taste and in the feeling of satiety, which can have a significant role in altering eating behaviors.[9]

Olfactory Flavor

The appreciation of flavor requires an integration of somatosensory and chemesthetic sensation from the oral cavity and oropharynx and intact retronasal olfaction. Chewing warms and releases odors, and the pressure changes created by swallowing pumps the odors through the oral pharynx and nasopharynx to the olfactory epithelium.[2] Duffy and colleagues[3] have shown that, when compared with young subjects, elderly individuals required 49 times the concentration of olfactory flavoring for consistent detection. This loss of olfactory flavor is consistent with the decrease in olfactory function previously described; however, conditions in the mouth may affect retronasal olfaction and the appreciation of flavor independent of olfactory thresholds. Duffy and colleagues showed that dentures that cover the palate impede olfactory flavor sensitivity even with normal olfactory (smell) sensitivity. It is thought that this effect may be due to interference with normal chewing and mouth movements and may affect the mechanics of odor propagation up to the olfactory cleft. Oral cavity health is another variable when one considers the many etiologies of smell loss and the impact on the health and nutrition of the elderly.

PALLIATION OF SMELL LOSS IN THE NONELDERLY PATIENT

The management of smell loss in nonelderly patients can be frustrating for patients and care givers alike. Patients with nasal sinus disease have historically been the only subgroup of anosmic patients who have responded somewhat favorably to treatment. Patients with smell loss due to trauma, surgery, or viral disease have been more difficult to treat. Understanding prognostic data is essential in counseling this group of patients. Reden and colleagues[36] in a recent study reported on a large number of patients who had either posttraumatic or virally induced smell loss. Only 10% of posttraumatic patients recovered some smell over an average 14-month period. The post viral patients did better, with 32% recovering. Duncan and Seiden showed that recovery in these two populations can continue over a 3- to 5-year period. In their smaller study they showed slight improvement in 35% of trauma patients and 67% of post upper respiratory infection patients, suggesting that recovery can continue for an extended period of time.[37] Doty and colleagues[38] showed that parosmia was also common in patients who had posttraumatic smell loss. The prevalence of parosmia decreased from 41.1% to 15.4% over an 8-year period. Age has a significant role in the ability of patients to recover their sense of smell, with older patients showing less tendency to recover no matter the etiology. The authors' nonpublished observations at the University of Connecticut Taste and Smell Center suggest that any testable sense of smell seen within 1 year of the inciting event is usually a good prognostic indicator for perceptible recovery, especially in the post viral smell loss population.

Patients with loss of smell from posttraumatic or viral causes must be counseled as to what to expect and how to protect themselves from harm. Gas detectors are recommended if any heating or home appliances run on natural gas. Information on where to purchase these detectors can be obtained from local gas companies. Patients must be counseled regarding food storage and should be asked to label leftovers with dates of storage so that they can dispose of them appropriately. These patients are also treated for any underlying allergic rhinitis, even if mild in nature, because this mild disease may impair their ability to appreciate any smell that does return.

SUMMARY

The decrease in smell sensitivity in the elderly has been well documented. The etiology of the loss of smell as a concomitant of the process of aging appears to be multifactorial and not entirely understood. Detecting and evaluating smell loss in this population can have a significant role in helping to maintain good nutrition and avoid food aversions.

REFERENCES

1. Mozaffarian D, Kumanyika SK, LeMaitre RN, et al. Fruit and vegetable fiber intake and the risk of cardiovascular disease in elderly individuals. J Am Med Assoc 2003;289:1659–66.
2. Duffy VB. Variation in oral sensation: implications for diet and health. Curr Opin Gastroenterol 2007;23:171–7.
3. Duffy VB, Cain WS, Ferris AM. Measurement of sensitivity to olfactory flavor: application in a study of aging and dentures. Chem Senses 1999;24:671–7.
4. Duncan HJ, Smith DV. Clinical disorders of olfaction. In: Doty RL, editor. Handbook of olfaction and gustation. New York: Marcel-Dekker; 1995. p. 345–65.
5. Nordin S, Monsch AU, Murphy C. Unawareness of smell loss in normal aging and Alzheimer's disease: discrepancy between self-reported and diagnosed smell sensitivity. J Gerontol B Psychol Sci Soc Sci 1995;50:187–92.

6. Smutzer GS, Doty RL, Arnold SE, et al. Olfactory system neuropathology in Alzheimer's disease, Parkinson's disease and schizophrenia. In: Doty RL, editor. Handbook of olfaction and gustation. New York: Marcel-Dekker; 2003. p. 503–23.

7. Rawson NE. Olfactory loss in aging. Sci Aging Knowledge Environ 2006;5:6.

8. Lewis LL, Dahl AR. Olfactory mucosa—composition, enzymatic localization, and metabolism. In: Doth RL, editor. Handbook of olfaction and gustation. New York: Marcel-Dekker; 1995. p. 33–52.

9. Luzzi S, Snowsen JS, Neary D, et al. Distinct patterns of olfactory impairment in Alzheimer's disease, semantic dementia, frontotemporal dementia, and cortico-basal degeneration. Neuropsychologia 2007;45:1823–31.

10. Robinson AM, Conley MD, Shinners MD, et al. Apoptosis in the aging olfactory epithelium. Laryngoscope 2002;112:1431–5.

11. Kern RC, Conley DB, Haines GK, et al. Pathology of the olfactory mucosa: implications for the treatment of olfactory dysfunction. Laryngoscope 2004;114:279–85.

12. Schemper T, Voss S, Cain WS. Odor identification in young and elderly persons: sensory and cognitive limitations. J Gerontol 1981;36(4):446–52.

13. Doty RL, Shaman P, Applebaum SL, et al. Smell identification ability: changes with age. Science 1984;226(4681):1441–3.

14. Stevens JC, Cain WS. Old-age deficits in the sense of smell as gauged by thresholds, magnitude matching and odor identification. Psychol Aging 1987;2:26–42.

15. Cain WS, Gent JF. Olfactory sensitivity: reliability, generality and association with aging. J Exp Psychol 1991;17:382–91.

16. de Wijk RA, Cain WS. Odor identification by name and by edibility: lifespan development and safety. Hum Factors 1994;36:182–7.

17. Leopold DA, Bartoshuk L, Doty RL, et al. Aging of the upper airway and the senses of taste and smell. Otolaryngol Head Neck Surg 1989;100(4):287–9.

18. Doty RL, Shaman P, Dann M. Development of the University of Pennsylvania smell identification test: a standardized microencapsulated test of olfactory function. Physiol Behav 1984;32(3):489–502.

19. Cain WS, Goodspeed RB, Gent J, et al. Evaluation of olfactory dysfunction in the Connecticut Chemosensory Research Center. Laryngoscope 1988;98(1):83–8.

20. Murphy C, Schubert CR, Cruikshanks KJ, et al. Prevalence of olfactory impairment in older adults. J Am Med Assoc 2002;288:2307–12.

21. Ferry M. Strategies for ensuring good hydration in the elderly. Nutr Rev 2005;63: S22–9.

22. Antunes MB, Bowler R, Doty RL. San Francisco/Oakland Bay Bridge welder study. Neurology 2007;69(12):1278–84.

23. Gobba F. Olfactory toxicity: long-term effects of occupational exposures. Int Arch Occup Environ Health 2006;79:322–31.

24. Nakashima T, Kimmelman CP, Snow JB. Structure of human fetal and adult olfactory neuroepithelium. Arch Otolaryngol 1984;110:641–6.

25. Rosli Y, Breckenridge LJ, Smith RA. An ultrastructural study of age-related changes in mouse olfactory epithelium. J Electron Microsc 1999;48(1):77–84.

26. Vent J, Robinson AM, Gentry-Nielsen MJ, et al. Pathology of the olfactory epithelium: smoking and ethanol exposure. Laryngoscope 2004;114:1383–8.

27. Rawson NE, Gomez G, Cowart B, et al. The use of olfactory receptor neurons (ORNs) from biopsies to study changes in ageing and neurodegenerative diseases. Ann N Y Acad Sci 1998;855:701–7.

28. Loo AT, Youngentob SL, Kent PF, et al. The aging olfactory epithelium: neurogenesis, response to damage, and odorant-induced activity. Int J Dev Neurosci 1996; 14(7–8):881–900.

29. Christensen MD, Holbrook EH, Costanzo RM, et al. Rhinotopy is disrupted during re-innervation of the olfactory bulb that follows transection of the olfactory nerve. Chem Senses 2001;26:359–69.
30. Bhatnagar KP, Kennedy RC, Baron G, et al. Number of mitral cells and the bulb volume in the aging human olfactory bulb: a quantitative morphological study. Anat Rec 1987;218:73–87.
31. Attems J, Lintner F, Jellinger KA. Olfactory involvement in aging and Alzheimer's disease: an autopsy study. J Alzheimers Dis 2005;7:149–57.
32. Masaoka Y, Yoshimura N, Inoue M, et al. Impairment of odor recognition in Parkinson's disease caused by weak activations of the orbitofrontal cortex. Neuroscience Lett 2007;412:45–50.
33. Tsuboi Y, Wszolek ZK, Graff-Radford NR, et al. Tau pathology in the olfactory bulb correlates with Braak stage, Lewy body pathology and apolipoprotein E4. Neuropathol Appl Neurobiol 2003;29:503–10.
34. Braak H, Braak E. Neuropathological stageing of Alzheimer-related changes. Acta Neuropathol 1991;82(4):239–59.
35. Kovacs T. Mechanisms of olfactory dysfunction in aging and neurodegenerative disorders. Aging Res Rev 2004;3:215–32.
36. Reden J, Mueller A, Konstantinidis I, et al. Recovery of olfactory function following closed head injury or infections of the upper respiratory tract. Arch Otolaryngol Head Neck Surg 2006;132(3):265–9.
37. Duncan HJ, Seiden AM. Long term follow up of olfactory loss secondary to head trauma and upper respiratory tract infection. Arch Otolaryngol Head Neck Surg 1995;121(10):1183–7.
38. Doty RL, Yousem DM, Pham LT, et al. Olfactory dysfunction in patients with head trauma. Arch Archives of Neurology 1997;54(9):1131–40.

Tracheostomy in Palliative Care

Teresa Chan, MD[a], Anand K. Devaiah, MD, FACS[a,b],*

KEYWORDS

- Tracheostomy • Palliation • Respiratory failure • Ventilator
- ALS • End of life • Aspiration

Tracheostomy is a procedure with a long history. The earliest account of tracheostomy is depicted in Egyptian tablets dating back around 3600 BC.[1] Although other accounts from Egypt and India describe what are believed to be tracheostomy procedures, a formally recognized account of elective tracheostomy is credited to Aesclepiades of Bithynia in the first century BC. The earliest accounts of tracheostomy largely described the procedure as a life-saving maneuver associated with a high mortality risk. Although early physicians such as Galen hailed the procedure as holding promise for patients, millennia would pass before the inherent risks could be overcome to make the procedure more acceptable.[2,3]

Pierre Bretonneau is credited as being one of the pioneers in making tracheostomy an accepted procedure. In the 1820s, he described the use of tracheostomy for treatment of obstructive diphtheria. The procedure had a 73% mortality rate, which was still an improvement over the overall mortality of diphtheria at the time.[2] Chevalier Jackson's pioneering work in laryngology and bronchoesophagology during the late 1800s helped to improve the tracheostomy procedure. His work in understanding and manipulating the airway helped improve the surgical techniques of tracheostomy to make it a safer procedure. Use of the procedure, particularly in the treatment of airway obstruction, became a more viable alternative with a lower mortality. The use of tracheostomy decreased with the development of a diphtheria antiserum. When cases of diphtheria dropped by the early 1900s, removing this disease as a significant health threat, the rate of tracheostomy decreased concomitantly.[4]

One could credit the ravages of polio and post polio syndrome as leading to the resurgence of tracheostomy and its consideration in palliative care. In 1928, the iron lung was successfully used on a pediatric patient with polio-induced respiratory failure.[5,6] As a noninvasive means of ventilation, this device was useful and saved

a Department of Otolaryngology—Head and Neck Surgery, Boston University School of Medicine, Boston Medical Center, D608 Collamore, 88 East Newton Street, Boston, MA 02118, USA
b Department of Neurological Surgery, Boston Medical Center, 88 East Newton Street, Boston, MA 02118, USA
* Corresponding author. Department of Otolaryngology—Head and Neck Surgery, Boston University School of Medicine, Boston Medical Center, D608 Collamore, 88 East Newton Street, Boston, MA 02118.
E-mail address: anand.devaiah@bmc.edu (A.K. Devaiah).

Otolaryngol Clin N Am 42 (2009) 133–141
doi:10.1016/j.otc.2008.09.002
0030-6665/08/$ – see front matter © 2009 Elsevier Inc. All rights reserved.
oto.theclinics.com

many lives; however, it was large and expensive, costing as much as the average home at the time. Such limitations led James Wilson to propose the use of tracheostomy in 1932 as a means of ventilation.[7] This consideration by Wilson helped moved tracheostomy from a treatment in obstruction to palliative ventilation.

ANATOMY AND SURGICAL TECHNIQUE

Knowledge of the relevant anatomy is important in tracheostomy. Although this anatomy is well known to those who perform the procedure, key elements are described herein for those who are less familiar. The trachea is palpable in the midline neck below the level of the thyroid cartilage and cricoid cartilage. Important landmarks to identify include the sternal notch, thyroid notch, thyroid cartilage, and cricoid cartilage. In patients with thick necks, intervening neck tumor, or life-threatening infection, the landmarks may be less prominent. The position of the thyroid gland is identified and is necessarily encountered in tracheostomy placement. One must be careful to identify these structures, because the trachea may be diverted off midline in some patients due to pathologic processes pushing the trachea to the side; in other patients the trachea may dive deep and away from the neck skin.

Tracheostomy may be performed by several means. The main divisions of tracheostomy methods are open and percutaneous. One version of the open method, preferred by the authors, is described briefly herein. The skin is palpated and marked below the level of the cricoid cartilage at the approximate level of the second tracheal ring. With the patient's neck extended using a shoulder roll and the skin prepared in a sterile fashion, a horizontal incision is made long enough to facilitate access to the deeper tissues and trachea. Once the strap muscles are encountered, they are pulled laterally after division of the median raphe. The thyroid isthmus is encountered and divided. The trachea is identified, and the interspace between the second and third tracheal rings is located (**Fig. 1**A). In any airway surgery clear communication with the anesthesia team is maintained because they need to assist in completing a successful tracheostomy without losing the airway. This interspace is sharply incised, and the trachea is entered.

Once the airway is entered, the final steps to creating a tract are at hand. For a long-term tracheostomy, it is recommended that a skin-trachea flap be developed. This flap allows for rapid creation of a well-defined tract and permits easy tracheostomy tube exchange in the short and long term. A common method is a Bjork flap. By making an inferiorly based U-shaped flap in the trachea, the skin is sutured down to this flap to create a tract (**Fig. 1**B). Another method is to remove a section of the trachea and suture the skin to the edges of the trachea circumferentially (**Fig. 1**C). Both of these methods can be particularly helpful in the palliative care setting in which a family member, visiting nurse, or nursing home practitioner primarily cares for the tracheostomy on a regular basis. After creating the opening and tract, an appropriately sized tracheostomy tube is placed within the opening and secured to the patient (**Fig. 2**). The authors prefer to suture the flanges to the skin and place a tracheostomy tie around the neck at the time of surgery.

The percutaneous method respects the same anatomic boundaries as in the open method. The airway is entered by first making a small skin incision. Concurrent tracheobronchoscopy to visualize the percutaneous airway instrumentation may be performed to reduce complications.[8] A needle is used to enter the tracheal interspace. Through the needle, a wire is passed in to the airway, which allows for percutaneous dilators to pass into the trachea. In this manner, the airway tract is developed for placing a tracheostomy tube.

There is an ongoing discussion over the merits of each method. Extensive review of this discussion is beyond the scope of this text; the notes provided in the following

A   **B**   **C**

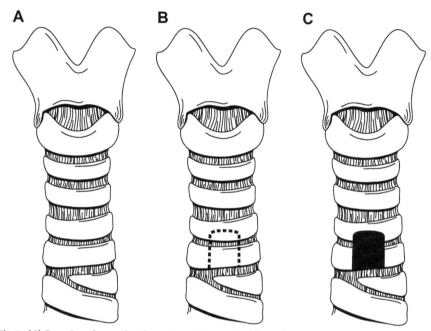

Fig.1. (*A*) Drawing shows the thyroid cartilage, cricoid cartilage, and upper rings of the trachea. (*B*) An inferior-based tracheal flap can be developed to sew to the skin and form a stable opening. This flap will open into the trachea and allow for passage of a tracheostomy
tube. (*C*) Alternatively, a segment of cartilage can be removed, allowing circumferential
sewing of skin to the edges of the tracheal opening.

sections are offered as general considerations. Each method has its advantages and
disadvantages. The open method allows for excellent visualization and creation of
a stable tract. Generally, it requires an operating room setting but can be performed
at the bedside with the proper set-up. The percutaneous method is facile at the
bedside and in the operating room. It should not be performed in patients who have
thick necks or distorted cervical anatomy, because there is increased risk of airway
and cervical complications. Both methods carry the risk of airway loss, bleeding,
trauma to the airway, and other complications. When compared with the earliest
efforts at the procedure, the surgery is generally safe and well tolerated by patients.

INDICATIONS AND DECISION MAKING IN PALLIATIVE CARE

The indications for tracheostomy as part of a palliative care plan do not differ greatly
from those in the acute or intensive care setting; however, the decision is often guided
by a different set of objectives, such as symptom relief, improvement in patient well-
being, facilitation of activities of daily living, and, if possible, optimization of long-term
function. Surgical intervention is not decided on the basis of curative outcomes which
are for the most part measurable and objective; instead, the decision must address
the foreseeable and imminent course of a patient's disease and take into account
other more humanistic factors such as spiritual needs and psychosocial resources.
Whenever tracheostomy is considered in the setting of palliative care, it is necessary
to have a dialogue about the patient's desire for his or her quality of life, their projected
prognosis, and the optimal timing in the natural progression of their disease.

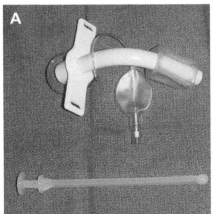
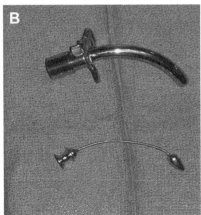
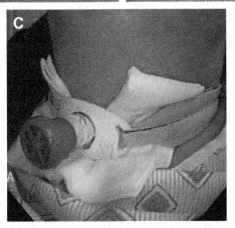

Fig. 2. Tracheostomy tubes come in a variety of types, such as cuffed plastic (A) and low-profile metal (B). (C) Shown is the appearance of a patient's neck in which dwells a well-healed tracheostomy site with a tracheostomy tube in place. At the end of this tube is a valve that allows for vocalization.

Of utmost importance is preservation of the quality of life. What this means may differ widely from patient to patient. In the setting of terminal illness, this discussion naturally extends into the topic of the quality of dying as well. Patients and their families are often concerned about the potential limitations that tracheostomy and eventual ventilator dependence will place on the patient's quality of life.[9] Often, there are concerns that tracheostomy serves to prolong life without contributing significantly to quality of life.[10] Additionally, for most patients, a tracheostomy implies an impending change in swallowing and speech function. It is necessary for the physician to address these fears, to present possible options for voice and swallowing preservation, and to discuss realistic outcomes for the individual patient before proceeding. In the setting of progressive motor neuron or neuromuscular disease, this conversation is often complicated by the anticipated decline in bulbar function which was perhaps the impetus for discussion of tracheostomy in the first place. Early involvement of a speech and language pathology team may be helpful in optimizing long-term outcomes.

Tracheostomy should be considered in the context of a patient's desires and beliefs and integrated as part of a larger long-term palliative care plan. If needed and timed properly, it can contribute greatly to the quality of a patient's life.

Common reasons for placement of a tracheostomy include airway obstruction, chronic aspiration, or the need for pulmonary toilet or prolonged ventilation from general deconditioning, an acute neural insult, or progressive neuromuscular decline. Loss of control of any one of the closely coordinated functions of the upper aerodigestive tract (respiration, deglutition, or speech) often may result in difficulties with the others. Each of these indications is discussed herein with particular attention to relevant issues in palliative care.

Airway Obstruction or Prolonged Ventilation

The need to secure an airway in the setting of impending airway compromise seems at first glance to require little discussion. Examples of possible airway obstruction encountered in the palliative care setting include unresectable malignancies of the oral cavity, oropharynx, larynx, and thyroid; vocal cord fixation from invasive tracheal tumors; and obstructive cervical metastases. In addition to obstructive processes, decline in muscular control of the upper aerodigestive tract or generalized deconditioning may necessitate long-term mechanical ventilation and intubation.

In the setting of palliative care when impending airway obstruction or compromise may not be on the order of minutes but projected on the order of weeks to months, anticipation is key. As Ross and Abrahm advocate in their article,[11] discussion of palliative surgery should ideally happen on a continuum of disease management rather than when the patient reaches the point of distress or extremis. This dialogue should be an ongoing and paced discussion that anticipates but does not unduly burden the patient or family physically, psychologically, socially, or spiritually.

Symptom anticipation is an advanced approach to the principle of symptom management in palliative care. Anticipatory management before catastrophic events is desirable and supported by outcomes. There is a greater complication rate with emergency airway management in the field and in the hospital.[12,13] Cricothyroidotomy carries with it the highest risk of complication, ranging from 13% to 40%.[12] Elective tracheostomy has about a 15% complication rate, and emergency tracheostomy is estimated to be associated with two to five times the risk of elective tracheostomy.[12] Moreover, within a hospital setting, cricothyroidotomy was successful in only 87% of attempts to establish an airway, whereas tracheostomy was successful in securing the airway in 100% of attempts.[12] In the field, the adequacy of cricothyroidotomy decreased to 64%, but this was not recognized until arrival at a trauma center. In fact, advanced life support providers judged that they had adequately secured these airways via cricothyroidotomy in 89% of patients.[13]

The primary physician responsible for coordinating the patient's palliative care plan should engage the patient, family members, and appropriate consultants in an interdisciplinary dialogue early in the onset of disease. This collaboration may include disease specialists such as oncologists, surgeons, anesthesiologists, speech language pathologists, nurses, social workers, and clergy. This discussion should ideally occur when airway compromise is foreseen as the natural course of disease, before the point when the urgency of the decision obscures the ability to weigh the patient's values and desires adequately. The discussion of tracheostomy should be integrated as a part of an ongoing discussion of the patient's long-term plan rather than a separate singular surgical intervention. The patient should be presented with any reasonable alternatives for airway management, such as surgical debulking of a tumor or palliative radiation and chemotherapy with the goal of relieving tumor burden.

Ultimately, the decision for or against tracheostomy should be left to the patient; however, specialists and primary palliative care providers have the obligation to ensure that a patient understands the ramifications of his or her decisions. For instance, a patient with an unresectable cancer of the upper aerodigestive tract who refuses tracheostomy as part of their care plan must understand what he or she is choosing in terms of comfort and dignity in dying by progressive respiratory compromise.

Chronic Aspiration and the Need for Pulmonary Toilet

Chronic aspiration and pulmonary toilet requirements are common, closely related indications for tracheostomy in palliative care. Loss of specific muscle coordination due to decline of bulbar function, loss of lower cranial nerves secondary to stroke, the mass effect or fixation of any part of the swallowing apparatus from a sizable head and neck tumor, excessive gastric secretions in gastrointestinal cancers or carcinomatosis of the bowel, and general deconditioning are all situations that may predispose a patient to chronic aspiration and the need for aggressive pulmonary toilet.

Tracheostomy should not be thought of as a cure for aspiration. In fact, tracheostomy can worsen aspiration by preventing elevation of the larynx with swallowing. Schonhofer and colleagues[14] reported a 30% aspiration rate in patients who were tracheotomized.

First-line measures for the prevention of aspiration include pharmacologic control of excessive secretions, limitation of food consistencies based on swallow evaluation, reinforcement of swallowing techniques by a speech language pathologist, and the use of nonoral feeding options (eg, parenteral nutrition and nasogastric tube feeds). If all other medical alternatives have been attempted and deemed ineffective for a long-term solution, consideration of surgical management options including tracheostomy is appropriate. In the palliative care setting, surgical intervention may be justified for intractable life-threatening aspiration and on the basis of improving patient comfort.

CONTRAINDICATIONS

The most obvious contraindication to tracheostomy or any surgical intervention is patient objection. Both a patient's conscious objection and his or her inability to knowingly consent to the procedure should be reason to stop and seek alternatives. Although preservation of patient autonomy is the most basic tenet taught from the first years of medical school, it can be disconcerting to a physician when a patient's decision contradicts what would be thought of as "the best option" medically speaking. In palliative care as in all health care circumstances, the patient's right to decide must be respected and upheld.

Establishment of advanced directives and a proxy decision maker before cognitive decline is desirable and the current standard of practice. Nevertheless, observations from the SUPPORT study found that many patients would not want their prehospitalization resuscitation preferences strictly followed if they were to lose decision-making capacity. They would prefer their family and physician to make resuscitation decisions for them.[15]

Other relative contraindications to tracheostomy include anatomic or patient factors that preclude safe effective tracheostomy with an acceptable blood loss. For example, in the situation of a large thyroid malignancy that obscures safe surgical access to the airway, it may be in the patient's best interest to remain intubated rather than undergo tracheostomy. In the situation of an obstruction distal to the trachea for which the patient remains chronically intubated (eg, obstructing lymphoma of a mainstem bronchus), tracheostomy would be of little help in ventilation. If a patient's belief system precludes the use of adjuncts that might be necessary for safe surgery, one must proceed with caution to surgical intervention. Anesthetic factors such as pulmonary reserve, cardiac health, and expected blood loss in the setting of bleeding diatheses are all risks that must be weighed against the benefits of surgery.

Ultimately, when deciding whether to operate, three questions should be asked and answered: (1) Does the patient understand and desire this intervention and its alternatives? (2) Will this intervention facilitate palliation or supportive care? (3) Do the benefits of the procedure outweigh the risks?

USE OF TRACHEOSTOMY IN PALLIATIVE CARE

Progressive neuromuscular or motor neuron disease can lead to any of the previously listed indications for tracheostomy, and much of the current literature about end-of-life use comes from studies of patients with amyotrophic lateral sclerosis (ALS).[16–18] For this subset of palliative care patients, the use and optimal timing of tracheostomy is possibly the most controversial. Without some form of respiratory support, the current 5-year survival rate for patients with ALS is approximately 7% to 20%, with a median survival of 19 to 30 months from diagnosis.[19,20] Many of these patients are able to function comfortably with noninvasive ventilation (non-assisted ventilation with nasal prongs for oxygen supplementation) for a time, especially if bulbar involvement has been spared; however, if bulbar impairment is more severe or if noninvasive ventilation is not tolerated, a tracheostomy and positive pressure ventilation are sometimes sought.

Despite the survival statistics, the overall rate of use of tracheostomy and mechanical ventilation in patients with ALS or other motor neuron diseases is low in the United States, approximately 4% or less.[18] This rate is consistent with the overall pattern of resource use in this subset of patients. In a study by Albert and colleagues,[18] a total of 121 ALS patients were followed up for a median of 12 months. Twenty-two percent had percutaneous gastrostomy (PEG), 19.4% used Bi-PAP, and 4.3% had a tracheostomy. Many patients did not take advantage of palliative care options before death. For example, 36.6% used hospice, 48% had signed a power of attorney form, and 18% had "do not resuscitate" orders in their medical charts. The reasons are not completely clear, although many explanations have been sought.

In a 1999 article by Albert which looked at preferences and actual treatment choices in ALS patients, initial preferences toward tracheostomy and PEG tube placement coincided with the eventual treatment choices. Patients who found the interventions initially acceptable and who went on to use them were more likely to be recently diagnosed, expressed a greater attachment to life, and showed great declines in pulmonary function over follow-up.[16] A separate article investigating the incidence and predictors of PEG placement in patients with ALS and other motor neuron diseases corroborates these data. The strongest predictor for PEG use was the patient's baseline preference, and patients who were inclined to PEG tubes were also more likely to be proactive in their own care and to have established health care proxies in advance. Patients who received PEG were also more likely to have tracheostomies than patients not using PEG.[17]

In a study by Rabkin, 72 hospice-eligible ALS patients were followed up until tracheostomy or death. Fourteen patients, nearly 20%, chose long-term mechanical ventilation and 58 died without it. The profile of the patients who chose tracheostomy was as follows: younger patients with more young children, more education, and higher household incomes on average. Although their physical conditions were similar, they reported higher levels of optimism, including a belief in imminent cure and more positive appraisals of their ability to function in daily life, their physical health, and overall life satisfaction. At study entry, none of the patients who later chose tracheostomy and long-term ventilation were clinically depressed compared with 26% of those who ultimately refused tracheostomy.[10]

ALS patients are a special subset of palliative care patients. They are typically young and healthy before diagnosis and experience rapid functional decline over 1 to 5 years. Although they are faced with similar dilemmas in end-of-life care as older patients or those with chronic disease, any broad conclusions about palliative care patients with respect to tracheostomy or other considerations from the perspective of this unique subset of patients should be drawn with caution.

The timing of the discussion of tracheostomy and the circumstances of the decision also influence the likelihood of a patient electing to undergo tracheostomy. Whether this occurs in the acute care/intensive care setting, outpatient, or post intensive care setting influences the gravity of the situation and the perceived prognosis. In a study by Lloyd and colleagues[21] looking at intensive care decision making in the seriously ill and elderly, 50 patients were followed up prospectively. Seriously ill patients were defined as adult inpatients with chronic illness and an estimated 50% 6-month mortality rate. Also included in the study were patients aged 80 years and older with an acute illness. Patients were given two options: (1) mechanical ventilation for 14 days or (2) mechanical ventilation for 1 month followed by placement of a tracheostomy and feeding tube. There was a wide variation in the preference for aggressive care that did not appear to be influenced by the prehospitalization quality of life. The predicted quality of life appeared to be as important as estimates of intensive care unit survival in decision making. When confronted with extended mechanical ventilation and associated care, a significant proportion of patients would accept this care only for an improved prognosis.

FUTURE DIRECTIONS

Although the surgical method of tracheostomy is less likely to have marked enhancements, gains may be realized in other areas such as the decision-making process. We can further hone the tenets of medical ethics, further stratify risk (both short and long term), and refine our understanding of overall patient benefits. The gain is in maximizing judicious use of palliative tracheostomy. To arrive at this without compromising long-term outcomes while improving the quality of remaining life would be highly desirable.

On the less esoteric side, further improvements in tracheostomy cannulas may bring benefits. By refining the assortment of airway cannulas that allow for a stable airway, proper ventilation, good pulmonary toilet, and low material complications, patient benefit can be increased. Accidental decannulation due to excessive mobility or poor placement/replacement of the cannula still occurs and can be devastating. Further developments in cannula design to reduce interference in speech production and swallowing are other areas for improvement. In palliative patients who have other upper aerodigestive tract compromise, the airway cannula can be a lifesaver and a detriment to their remaining quality of life.

SUMMARY

The use of tracheostomy in palliative care offers a viable option for airway control. Through a dialogue with the patient, family, and a multidisciplinary set of providers, this procedure can be a useful component to a patient's overall palliative care plan.

REFERENCES

1. Pahor AL. Ear, nose, and throat in ancient Egypt. J Laryngol Otol 1992;106(9): 773–9.
2. The early history of the tracheostomy. 2007. Available at: http://www.entlink.net/museum/exhibits/Early-History.cfm. Accessed November 1, 2007.
3. Stock CR. What is past is prologue: a short history of the development of the tracheostomy. Ear Nose Throat J 1987;66(4):166–9.
4. Standardization and alternate methods of tracheostomy. 2007. Available at: http://www.entlink.net/museum/exhibits/trach_alternatives.cfm. Accessed November 1, 2007.
5. Graamans K, Pirsig W, Biefel K. The shift in indications for the tracheostomy between 1940 and 1955: an historical review. J Laryngol Otol 1999;113(7):624–7.
6. Branson RD. A tribute to John H. Emerson. Jack Emerson: notes on his life and contributions to respiratory care. Respir Care 1998;43(7):567–71.
7. Wilson JL. Acute anterior poliomyelitis: treatment of bulbar and high spinal types. N Engl J Med 1932;206:887–93.
8. Tomsic JP, Connolly MC, Joe VC, et al. Evaluation of bronchoscopic-assisted percutaneous tracheostomy. Am Surg 2006;72(10):970–2.
9. Bach JR. A comparison of long-term ventilatory support alternatives from the perspective of the patient and care giver. Chest 1993;104(6):1702–6.
10. Rabkin JG, Albert SM, Tider T, et al. Predictors and course of elective long-term mechanical ventilation: a prospective study of ALS patients. Amyotroph Lateral Scler 2006;7(2):86–95.
11. Ross EL, Abrahm J. Preparation of the patient for palliative procedures. Surg Clin North Am 2005;85(2):191–207.
12. Gillespie MB, Eisele DW. Outcomes of emergency surgical airway procedures in a hospital-wide setting. [Triological Society Papers]. Laryngoscope 1999; 109(11):1766–9.
13. Fortune JB, Judkins DG, Scanzaroli D, et al. Efficacy of prehospital surgical cricothyroidotomy in trauma patients. J Trauma 1997;42:832–6.
14. Schonhofer B, Barchfeld T, Haidl P, et al. Scintigraphy for evaluating early aspiration after oral feeding in patients receiving prolonged ventilation via tracheostomy. Intensive Care Med 1999;25(3):311–4.
15. Puchalski CM, Zhong Z, Jacobs MM, et al. Patients who want their family and physician to make resuscitation decisions for them: observations from Support and Help. Study to Understand Prognoses and Preferences for Outcomes and Risks of Treatment: Hospitalized Elderly Longitudinal Project. J Am Geriatr Soc 2000;48:S84–90.
16. Albert SM, Murphy PL, Del Bene ML, et al. A prospective study of preferences and actual treatment choices in ALS. Neurology 1999;53:278.
17. Albert SM, Murphy PL, Del Bene M, et al. Incidence and predictors of PEG placement in ALS/MND. J Neurol Sci 2001;191(1–2):115–9.
18. Albert SM, Murphy PL, Del Bene ML, et al. Prospective study of palliative care in ALS: choice, timing, outcomes. J Neurol Sci 1999;169(1–2):108–13.
19. Del Aguila MA, Longstreth WT Jr, McGuire V, et al. Prognosis in amyotrophic lateral sclerosis: a population-based study. Neurology 2003;60(5):813–9.
20. Millul A, Beghi E, Logroscino G, et al. Survival of patients with amyotrophic lateral sclerosis in a population-based registry. Neuroepidemiology 2005;25(3):114–9.
21. Lloyd CB, Nietert PJ, Silvestri GA. Intensive care decision making in the seriously ill and elderly. Crit Care Med 2004;32(3):649–54.

Alleviating Head and Neck Pain

Abdel-Kader Mehio, MD*, Swapneel K. Shah, MD

KEYWORDS

- Cervicogenic headache • Interventional procedures
- Malignancy • Radiofrequency • Ablation

The great humanitarian, physician, and Nobel Laureate Albert Schweitzer described the nature of pain and the obligation and privilege that a physician holds to try and relieve it. Referring to the duty of physicians, he stated, "We must all die. But that I can save him from days of torture, that is what I feel as my great and ever new privilege. Pain is a more terrible lord of mankind than even death itself."[1] Practitioners treating pain, as it relates to the head and neck, can relate to the concerns of Dr. Schweitzer. Many of their patients suffer pain as a result of malignancies. Head and neck cancer accounts for 5% to 10% of malignant tumors, and the cure rate of tumors of the head and neck region is only 35%. Pain is a presenting symptom in 20% of patients having tumors of the oral cavity and is experienced by 40% to 80% of patients having head and neck cancer. These patients are not only coming to grips with their increased likelihood of death but also with the potential for pain and the possibility of impairment of such simple functions as swallowing and breathing. Another common but potentially debilitating cause of head pain is cervical spine abnormalities, which cannot only produce neck pain but cervicogenic headache as well.

Pain in patients who have cancer can be caused by direct effects of the tumor (eg, invasion of bone by tumor, nerve compression) or by complications of treatment (eg, radiation fibrosis, chemotherapy-induced neuropathy), or it can be unrelated to the disease or its treatment. The aggressive use of pharmacologic treatments (nonsteroidal anti-inflammatory drugs [NSAIDS], opioids, antidepressants, muscle relaxants, anticonvulsants, α_2-receptor agonists, corticosteroids, and bisphosphonates) is generally successful.[2] When effective pain relief cannot be achieved by these modalities, however, specialized interventional approaches may offer an alternative. These include (1) intraspinal analgesia (opioids and local anesthetics), which is the most commonly used approach; (2) neurosurgical techniques (eg, cordotomy, rhizotomy, dorsal root entry zone lesioning [DREZ], hypophysectomy), most of which involve severing a component of the nerve conduction pathway involved in pain; (3) nonsurgical interventional procedures, including sympathetic and somatic nerve blocks in addition to localized

Department of Anesthesiology, Boston Medical Center, 88 East Newton Street, Boston, MA 02118, USA
* Corresponding author.
E-mail address: amehio@bu.edu (A-K. Mehio).

Otolaryngol Clin N Am 42 (2009) 143–159
doi:10.1016/j.otc.2008.09.013
0030-6665/08/$ – see front matter © 2009 Elsevier Inc. All rights reserved.

injections of anesthetic agents with or without steroids, and radiofrequency ablation and nonablation procedures. This topic emphasizes the application of some interventional pain procedures in the treatment of head and neck.

MECHANISMS OF PAIN
Cervicogenic

The zygapophysial joint, also known as a facet joint, is a synovial joint between the superior articular process of one (lower) vertebra and the inferior articular process of the adjacent (higher) vertebra. There are two facet joints in each vertebral motion segment (**Fig. 1**). The biomechanical function of each pair of facet joints is to prevent excessive torsion (twisting) of the spine, although allowing a small amount of lateral bending and flexion and extension. As with any synovial joint degeneration, inflammation and injury can lead to pain on joint motion. Restriction of motion secondary to pain can lead to overall physical deconditioning, and irritation of the joint innervation can itself lead to secondary muscle spasm.

It has long been proposed, and more recently accepted, that cervical spine structures, particularly those innervated by the upper three cervical nerves, have the capacity to refer pain into the head and cause neck pain and headache.[3–6] The anatomic substrate for this referred head pain is the trigeminal nucleus.[3] Anatomically, any nociceptive activity arising from disease or disorders in upper cervical joint structures (ie, zygapophysial joints, C0–C3), in muscles innervated by the upper three cervical nerves, or in the nerves themselves can access the trigeminal nucleus, and thus can be responsible for headache.[3]

Neurophysiologic and anatomic studies have found small-diameter high-threshold pain fibers in the zygapophysial joint capsules of humans and rabbits.[7,8] In addition, fibers containing several peptides associated with nociceptive transmission have been identified in the synovial folds of the facet joint.[9] Dwyer and colleagues[10] developed diagrams of cervical zygapophysial joint pain distribution in healthy volunteers by provocative injection (**Fig. 2**). Given the preponderance of clinical data, in addition to insight into the possible pathophysiologic basis, cervical facet joints are increasingly being implicated in degenerative and traumatic head, neck, and posterior shoulder pain.

Despite knowing for many decades that cervical structures can refer pain to the head, knowledge of cervicogenic headache have been slow to evolve. It was not until 1983 that Sjaastad and colleagues[11] put forward the hypothesis that cervical musculoskeletal disorders produced a distinct headache type, which they named "cervicogenic

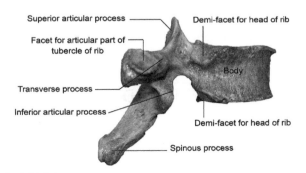

Superior articular process
Demi-facet for head of rib
Facet for articular part of tubercle of rib
Body
Transverse process
Inferior articular process
Demi-facet for head of rib
Spinous process

Fig. 1. Zygapophysial joint.

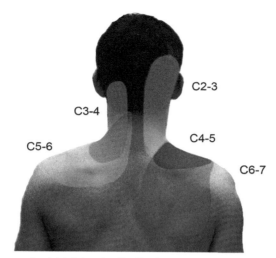

Fig. 2. Cervical zygapophysial joint pain distribution.

headache." In 1994, the International Association for the Study of Pain[6] was the first to accept the entity and classification of cervicogenic headache formally and to document the criteria for this headache type. With respect to the wider international community, it was not until 2004 that cervicogenic headache was provisionally accepted as a discrete headache type by the International Headache Society as published in their revised *International Classification of Headache Disorders* (ICHD-II).[11]

Malignancy

The mechanisms by which cancer can cause pain include (1) direct stimulation of nerve endings, (2) ulceration and infection, (3) compression and involvement of sensory nerves, and (4) bone invasion.[12] Nonnociception pain is also seen when nerve fibers exhibit abnormal excitatory patterns after being severed, which can be seen in patients who have undergone a neck dissection.[13]

Stimulation of nerve endings
Stimulation and sensitization of nociceptor nerve endings in the mucosa and submucosa are characteristic of the initial phases of cancer growth and can be considered to be mainly responsible for local burning sensation, superficial pain, and referred otalgia in exophytic or erosive lesions.[14]

Ulceration and infection
Most cancers that arise from the mucous membranes of the mouth and pharynx tend to ulcerate because of central necrosis and microtrauma. Ulceration does not produce spontaneous pain. Rather, pain is experienced after exposure to a local irritant agent, such as alcohol or acid, or after onset of infection with expression of inflammatory mediators. Movement markedly increases pain caused by ulceration, and its intensity varies from site to site. Exacerbation by functional activity is minimal in static regions, such as the cheek, hard palate, nasal and paranasal cavities, and nasopharynx. It is severe in dynamic structures, such as the tongue, floor of the mouth, soft palate, and faucial arches.[4]

Nerve compression and infiltration

An important cause of head and neck cancer pain is infiltration, compression, or both of one or more branches of the trigeminal nerve (CN V), glossopharyngeal nerve (CN IX), or other sensory cranial nerves (**Fig. 3**).

Bone invasion

Tumor involvement of bone is the most common cause of cancer pain.[15] Bone pain is purely somatic unless a pathologic fracture is present or tumor extension disrupts a nerve. The pain is usually described as focal and constant, although it may be referred to another site. Patients typically experience several days or weeks of increasing pain; acutely increased bone pain may signal a fracture or neural impingement. Locally, tumors may activate nociceptors by pressure, ischemia, or secretion of locally acting algesic substances (eg, prostaglandin E_2, osteoclast activating factor).[16] Most pain is probably sensed in the periosteum and synovium.

The cellular and neurochemical changes responsible for pain are incompletely identified. Cancer-related bone pain is caused by a tumor-induced imbalance between bone formation (mediated by osteoblasts) and resorption, which is mediated by osteoclasts. Osteoclasts resorb bone by secreting proteases that dissolve the matrix and by producing acid that releases bone mineral into the extracellular space.[17] The net result of this imbalance is bone destruction, which seems to be essential to the pathophysiology of bone cancer pain.[18]

PAIN SYNDROMES ASSOCIATED WITH MALIGNANCY OF THE HEAD AND NECK

Tumor involvement of the brain or surrounding skull can result in headache or facial pain, depending on the location and extent of tumor.

Headache

Patients who have cancer and experience new, different, or more frequent headaches should be investigated for brain metastases. Headache occurs in 60% of patients presenting with primary brain tumors and in 35% of those with cerebral metastases.

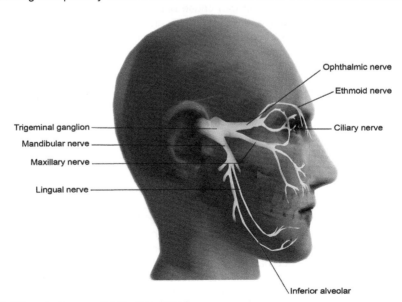

Fig. 3. Trigeminal nerve distribution (CN V).

The pain is usually of mild or moderate intensity, similar to a tension headache; only 25% of patients have awakening or morning headaches. Other associated symptoms and signs include nausea, vomiting, lethargy, photophobia, focal neurologic findings, mental status or personality changes, and sudden-onset (pressure-wave) and nocturnal headaches. The absence of these complaints does not rule out a brain tumor, however.

Multiple metastases, especially to the posterior fossa, and leptomeningeal carcinomatosis are the most frequent intracranial causes of headache. Other non–cancer-related causes include ischemic or hemorrhagic stroke, pseudotumor cerebri from superior vena cava syndrome, and sagittal sinus occlusion by tumor or thrombus.[19]

Headache may also result from traction, inflammation, or infiltration of the trigeminal, glossopharyngeal, vagus, accessory, or upper cervical nerves. The main dural arteries, dura mater, and tentorium cerebelli are also pain sensitive. Pain-sensitive extracranial structures include the galea, fascia, arteries, and muscles of the scalp.[20]

Facial Pain

Cancer is a rare cause of facial pain. Extracranial bony or soft tissue metastases may impinge on cranial and upper cervical nerves, causing headache or facial pain. Pain in these cases is less generalized, usually unilateral, and may be accompanied by focal tenderness. The following are some common facial pain syndromes in patients who have cancer:

- Tonsillar fossa tumors are frequently accompanied by pain that is at first mild and localized to the tonsil. As the tumor grows, however, pain becomes progressively more severe and spreads to the lateral wall of the pharynx and then to the entire distribution of the glossopharyngeal nerve. In the initial stages, the pain is some-what sharp, but as it spreads, it becomes more severe, continuous, persistent, dull, and aching and is accompanied by bouts of lancinating pain, referred otalgia, and generalized headache.
- Cancers of the maxillary antrum and upper jaw frequently produce pressure on branches of the maxillary nerve and, consequently, maxillary neuralgia, which is superimposed on the local pain caused by periosteal stretching and consequent stimulation of nociceptive endings.[4]
- Some tumors invade the pterygoid region and the infratemporal fossa and can involve the mandibular nerve or some of its branches to the muscle of mastication to produce neuralgia, trismus, and temporal pain. Tumors of the nasopharynx, oropharynx, or hypopharynx can compress and infiltrate branches of the glossopharyngeal and vagal nerves and produce neuralgia in their distribution in addition to localized pain.[4]

Atypical facial pain

Atypical facial pain can have many different causes, but the symptoms are all similar. By definition, it is persistent facial pain without the characteristics of cranial neuralgia and not attributable to another disorder (International Headache Society, 2004). Facial pain, often described as burning, aching, or cramping, typically occurs on one side of the face, often in the region of the trigeminal nerve, and can extend into the back of the scalp or upper neck. Although rarely as severe as trigeminal neuralgia, facial pain is continuous with rare periods of remission. The diagnosis is usually by process of elimination. A sphenopalatine ganglion block may be used therapeutically for chronic headaches or for atypical facial pain.

NERVE AND JOINT BLOCKS OF THE HEAD AND NECK

Several nerve block techniques are used in the management (therapeutic and diagnostic) of head and neck malignancy-associated pain. The same techniques can also be used to provide successful anesthesia and analgesia for a variety of procedures performed on the head and neck (**Table 1**).

TRIGEMINAL NERVE BLOCK
Indications

Trigeminal neuralgia is a rare form of neuropathic facial pain. Patients who have trigeminal neuralgia typically present with the spontaneous onset of pain in one or more divisions of the trigeminal nerve. The most common presentation involves V2 and V3, however, any or all divisions may be involved (**Fig. 4**). Patients report paroxysmal lancinating pain in the face that is often severe. The pain usually has a specific trigger point, and pressure on this trigger area elicits the pain.[21]

Anatomy and Technique

Lying at the apex of the petrous temporal bone at the junction of the middle and posterior cranial fossa, the gasserian ganglion is situated in a fold of dura mater that forms an invagination around its posterior two thirds. This invagination is a continuation of the cerebrospinal fluid (CSF) and is known as Meckel's cave or the cavum trigeminale.

The needle is placed through the skin 2 to 3 cm lateral to the lateral margin of the mouth and is advanced toward the mandibular condyle and toward the ipsilateral pupil until bone is contacted.[22] The needle is then withdrawn and redirected more posteriorly until the foramen ovale is entered.[22]

Table 1	
Nerve blocks of the head and neck	
Area of Pain	**Possible Nerve Block**
Head	
Face	Trigeminal nerve block
Orbit and contents, sphenoid sinus, eyelids, anterior two thirds of scalp	Ophthalmic nerve block
Forehead	Supraorbital nerve block
Upper jaw, maxillary antrum, distribution of infraorbital nerve	Maxillary nerve block
Lower eyelid, upper lip, temple, lateral aspect of the nose	Infraorbital nerve block
Lower jaw, teeth, anterior tongue, floor mouth	Mandibular nerve block, mental nerve block
Nose, palate	Sphenopalatine nerve block
Posterior third of tongue, soft palate, parotid gland	Glossopharyngeal nerve block
Neck	
Scalp, back of neck	Greater occipital nerve block
Shoulder and neck	Cervical plexus block, cervical paravertebral block, cervical epidural facet block
Larynx, trachea	Laryngeal nerve block, deep cervical plexus block

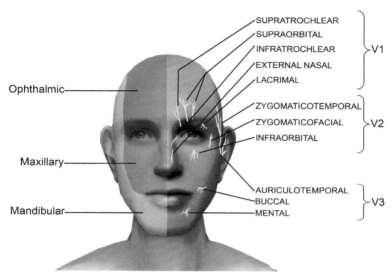

Fig. 4. Trigeminal nerve divisions.

SUPRAORBITAL AND SUPRATROCHLEAR NERVE BLOCKS
Indications

This block can produce analgesia of the forehead and scalp from the eyebrows to the vertex. This block can prove useful in conditions like Gradenigo-Lannois syndrome, which is caused by tumors involving the apex of the petrous temporal bone; secondary sarcomas of the base of the skull; meningioma; chondromas; neuroma of the gasserian ganglion and trigeminal root; and tumors of the pyramids. The pain is characteristically a frontal headache and neuralgia in the first (V1) and occasionally the second (V2) and third (V3) divisions of the trigeminal nerve.[5]

Anatomy and Technique

Both of these nerves, which emerge from within the orbit, are terminal divisions of the ophthalmic branch (V1) of the trigeminal nerve (CN V) (see **Fig. 4**). The supraorbital nerve emerges from the supraorbital foramen, which can be palpated along the upper border of the orbit, approximately 2.5 cm lateral to the midline of the face. The supraorbital nerve exits along the upper border of the orbit, approximately 1 cm medial to the supraorbital foramen. The supraorbital notch is palpated by the finger, and the needle is inserted along the upper orbital margin, approximately 1 cm medial to the supraorbital foramen, wherein 2 to 3 mL of local anesthetic is injected. The supratrochlear nerve, which emerges from the superomedial angle of the orbit, runs up on the forehead parallel to the supraorbital nerve a finger's breadth or so medial to it. This nerve is blocked as it emerges above the eyebrow or can be involved by a medial extension of the supraorbital block (**Fig. 5**).[13]

INFRATROCHLEAR AND ANTERIOR ETHMOIDAL NERVE BLOCK
Indications

The infratrochlear and anterior ethmoidal nerve block is used to provide analgesia of the nasal septum and the lateral wall of the nasal cavity.

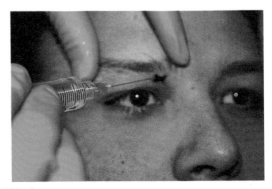

Fig. 5. Supraorbital block.

Anatomy and Technique

Sensation to the superior portions of the septum and lateral wall of the nasal cavity is supplied by the anterior ethmoidal nerve, a terminal branch of the V1 division of CN V (**Fig. 6**). The inferior and posterior portions of the septum and the lateral wall of the nasal cavity are innervated by branches arising from the sphenopalatine ganglion. These terminal branches lay superficially just beneath the nasal mucosa and can be anesthetized by direct topical application of local anesthetic.[23,24]

MAXILLARY NERVE BLOCK
Indications

As noted earlier, cancers of the maxillary antrum and upper jaw frequently produce pressure on branches of the maxillary nerve and, consequently, maxillary neuralgia,

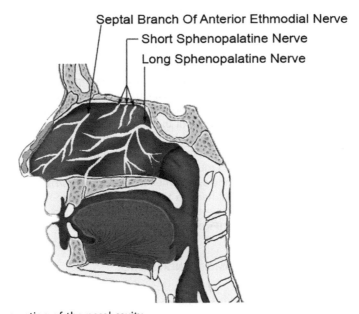

Septal Branch Of Anterior Ethmodial Nerve
Short Sphenopalatine Nerve
Long Sphenopalatine Nerve

Fig. 6. Innervation of the nasal cavity.

which is superimposed on the local pain caused by periosteal stretching and the consequent stimulation of nociceptive endings.[4] The block can provide analgesia of the upper jaw, maxillary antrum, and distribution of the infraorbital nerve.

Anatomy and Technique

The maxillary nerve is the V2 division of CN V (see **Fig. 4**). The nerve leaves the cranial cavity through the anterior wall of the middle cranial fossa by way of the foramen rotundum and traverses the pterygomaxillary fossa. The nerve is approached by way of the infratemporal fossa (by way of the coronoid notch below the midpoint of the zygoma). The needle passes through the infratemporal fossa to reach the lateral pterygoid plate.

The needle is then walked anteriorly until it passes into the pterygomaxillary fossa, where the maxillary nerve is located (**Fig. 7**).[13]

MANDIBULAR NERVE BLOCK
Indications

Some tumors invade the pterygoid region and the infratemporal fossa and can involve the mandibular nerve or some of its branches to the muscle of mastication to produce neuralgia, trismus, and temporal pain. Gasserian ganglion syndrome (middle fossa syndrome) is caused by a primary or metastatic lesion in the middle fossa and produces dysfunction of the gasserian ganglion or divisions of the trigeminal nerve. The pain and associated paresthesias are usually in the distribution of V2 and V3. The pain can be dull and aching in the cheek or jaw or lancinating (trigeminal neuralgia). Twenty-five percent of these patients also experience headaches.[5] A mandibular nerve block provides analgesia of the lower jaw, teeth, anterior tongue, and floor of the mouth. Kohase and colleagues[25,26] have described the application of a mandibular nerve block using an indwelling catheter for intractable cancer pain. They reported a case in which a mandibular nerve block utilizing an indwelling catheter was used for pain management in a terminal case of orofacial cancer.

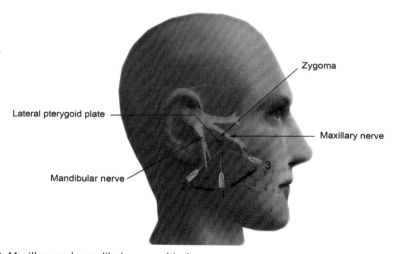

Fig. 7. Maxillary and mandibular nerve blocks.

Anatomy and Technique

The mandibular nerve is the V3 division of CN V (see **Fig. 4**). The largest branch of the trigeminal nerve, the mandibular branch, is sensory and motor. The sensory root arises from the trigeminal ganglion, whereas the motor root arises from the motor nucleus of the pons and medulla oblongata. The mandibular nerve gives off branches from its main trunk and from the anterior and posterior divisions.[14]

The approach for blocking the main division in the infratemporal fossa is the same, initially, as that described for the maxillary nerve; where it differs is that once the needle reaches the lateral pterygoid plate, it is walked posteriorly until a third-division paresthesia is obtained (see **Fig. 7**).[13]

GLOSSOPHARYNGEAL NERVE BLOCK
Indications

This block provides analgesia to the posterior third of tongue, soft palate, and parotid gland. As noted earlier, tonsillar fossa tumors are frequently accompanied by pain that is at first mild and localized to the tonsil; as the tumor grows, however, pain becomes progressively more severe and spreads to the lateral wall of the pharynx and then to the entire distribution of the glossopharyngeal nerve. This block is most frequently used for inoperable carcinomas that invade the distribution of the nerve in the posterior third of the tongue or the pharyngeal trapezius muscles.

Anatomy and Technique

The glossopharyngeal nerve (CN IX) emerges by way of the jugular foramen in relation to the vagus (CN X) and accessory (CN XI) nerves, along with the internal jugular vein. It is blocked just below this point; therefore, blocks usually involve all three cranial nerves, which lie in the groove between the internal jugular vein and internal carotid artery (**Fig. 8**). The needle is inserted at a point midway between the mastoid process and the angle of the mandible. At approximately 2 to 3 cm, the styloid process is contacted, and the needle is then walked posteriorly off the styloid process. Local anesthetic is injected at this point. In the 1970s, Cooper and Watson[27] and Funasaka and Kodera[28] described an alternative approach for intraorally blocking CN IX. Their technique involves injecting local anesthetic into the midpoint of the posterior pillar of the fauces (**Fig. 9**).

SUPERIOR LARYNGEAL NERVE AND RECURRENT LARYNGEAL NERVE BLOCKS
Indications

Blocks of the (internal) branch of the superior laryngeal nerve and the recurrent laryngeal nerve can render the laryngeal inlet and trachea insensitive to pain.

Anatomy and Technique

Both of these nerves are branches of CN X, the vagus nerve. The superior laryngeal nerve is blocked as it sweeps around the inferior border of the greater cornu of the hyoid bone (**Fig. 10**). This provides analgesia over the inferior aspect of the epiglottis and laryngeal inlet as far down as the vocal cords. Blockade of the recurrent laryngeal nerve produces analgesia below the cords. The simplest technique is by identifying and penetrating the cricothyroid membrane while the neck is extended (**Fig. 11**). After aspiration of air, local anesthetic is injected into the trachea at end expiration. A deep inhalation and cough immediately after injection distribute the anesthetic throughout the trachea.

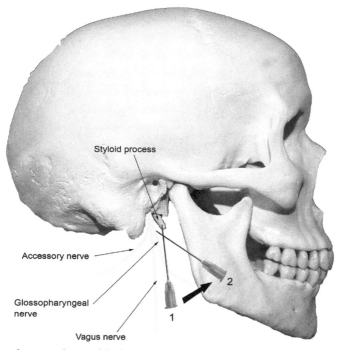

Styloid process

Accessory nerve

Glossopharyngeal
nerve

Vagus nerve

Fig. 8. Glossopharyngeal nerve block.

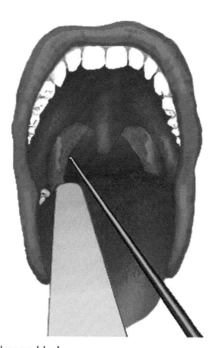

Fig. 9. Glossopharyngeal nerve block.

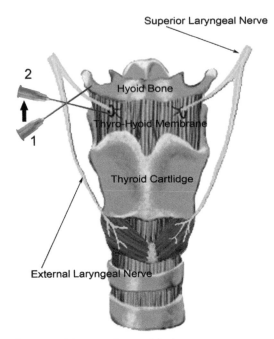

Fig. 10. Superior and recurrent laryngeal nerve blocks.

OCCIPITAL NERVE BLOCK
Indications

Occipital nerve block is most often used in the diagnosis and treatment of occipital neuralgia and cervicogenic headache. True occipital neuralgia typically follows blunt trauma to the nerves over the occiput and is characterized by pain in the distribution of the occipital nerves. Cervicogenic headache is more ill defined, insidious in onset, and characterized by pain in the same distribution. Many patients who have cervicogenic headaches have associated spondylosis of the cervical facet joints. When the pain is limited to the region overlying the occiput, occipital nerve blocks may be of some benefit in reducing the associated pain.[14]

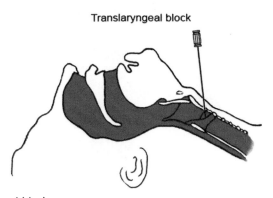

Fig. 11. Translaryngeal block.

Anatomy and Technique

The greater occipital nerve arises from the posterior primary ramus of the second cervical nerve root (**Fig. 12**). It travels deep to the cervical paraspinous musculature and becomes superficial just inferior to the superior nuchal line and lateral to the occipital protuberance of the skull. At this point, the nerve is just lateral to the occipital artery. The lesser occipital nerve and greater auricular nerve are terminal branches of the superficial cervical plexus. Both arise from the posterior primary ramus of the second and third cervical nerve roots, travel through the cervical paraspinous musculature, and become superficial over the inferior nuchal line of the skull, just superior and medial to the mastoid and just inferior to the tragus of the ear, respectively. The lateral section of the posterior scalp is supplied by the lesser occipital and great auricular nerves.[14]

For localization of the greater occipital nerve, the nerve is positioned medial to the pulse of the occipital artery, approximately one third of the distance from the occipital protuberance to the mastoid.

Pulsed Radiofrequency

In 1949, Hunter and Mayfield[4] described traumatic injury to the occipital nerves, which can cause occipital headaches. Treatment should be conservative initially and then interventional in the pain clinic in the form of occipital nerve blocks with local anesthetics and steroids. If unsuccessful, pulsed radiofrequency (PRF) is another option. It is a technique that uses an insulated needle to apply high voltage near the nerve but without the destructive effects of an increase in temperature. Because no injections are made, intravenous or intraneural injection of medication is not a concern.

Neuroaugmentation

Occipital nerve electrical stimulation is usually a last resort in patients who have intractable occipital neuralgia with debilitating headaches, and when other treatments have failed. A biphasic electrical pulse is applied by means of an electrode to the tissue surrounding the occipital nerve, a process that depolarizes the nerve and sends electrical impulses anterograde and retrograde through the nerve (**Fig. 13**). The result is an antinociceptive effect not only in the area innervated by the occipital nerve but in the

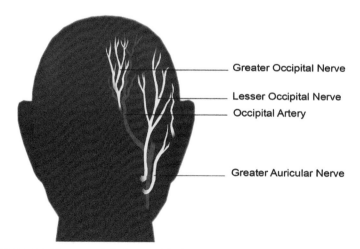

Greater Occipital Nerve

Lesser Occipital Nerve

Occipital Artery

Greater Auricular Nerve

Fig. 12. Greater and lesser occipital nerve block.

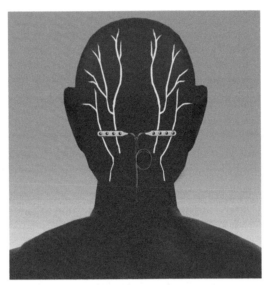

Fig. 13. Occipital nerve stimulation.

trigeminal distribution. Conditions like cluster headache, hemicrania continua, and migraine headache may improve with the application of this technique.

ZYGAPOPHYSIAL (FACET) JOINT BLOCK
Indications

As mentioned in previously, cervical facet joints are increasingly being implicated in degenerative and traumatic head, neck, and posterior shoulder pain in addition to cervicogenic headache. The available clinical data and insight into the possible pathophysiologic basis support the use of facet joint blocks in the management of these conditions.

Anatomy and Technique

The cervical zygapophysial joints below C2 to C3 are innervated by the medial branches of the dorsal rami of the spinal nerves above and below the joint.[28] Irritation of the medial branches could thus lead to generalized sensitization of the dorsal rami, with subsequent hyperactivity and spasm of the innervated muscles. The C2-to-C3 joint is supplied by the third occipital nerve. The medial branches travel across the waist of the articular pillar beneath the tendinous origin of the semispinalis capitis.

CERVICAL ARTICULAR BLOCKS

On the posterior neck, a needle is inserted at an angle of 45° to the skin and advanced to enter the joint or to contact the bony perimeter (**Fig. 14**). The appropriate skin entry site is two to three segments below the midpoint of the target joint. Adjustments are made under fluoroscopic view until the needle enters the joint capsule. Correct placement is confirmed with the injection of radiocontrast dye. Once needle placement is confirmed, the joint is injected with a mixture of local anesthetic and depot steroid.[29,30]

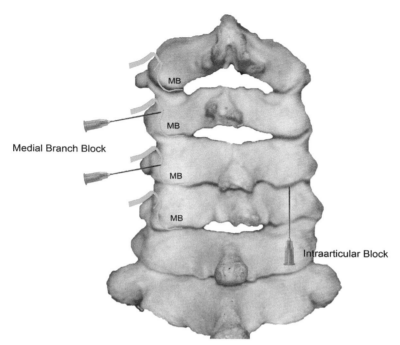

Fig. 14. Cervical zygapophysial joint blocks (medial branch & intra-articular).

CERVICAL MEDIAL BRANCH BLOCKS

The needle insertion site is just posterior to the carotid and jugular vessels, where the medial branch of the dorsal rami can be most easily reached. In this orientation, the articular pillar presents as a trapezoid, and the target point for C3 to C4 and lower levels is the centroid of the pillar (see **Fig. 14**). Care must be taken to avoid local anesthetic injection into the cervical nerve root and intravascular injection into the vertebral artery, which is anterior and medial to the needle target. For the C2-to-C3 level, the third occipital nerve is blocked at three evenly spaced locations along its course, bisecting the C3 articular pillar, usually with multiple injections sites because of its larger size and myelination pattern.

RADIOFREQUENCY ABLATION

Radiofrequency ablation is a method of localized hyperthermia resulting in tissue necrosis. Typically, an insulated needle with an active tip is introduced (usually under fluoroscopic guidance) to lie next to the target nerve. Heat is produced by the electric current and the nerve is ablated as such. Whereas tissue destruction begins at 45°C, the target temperature is approximately 80°C, which is applied for 60 to 90 seconds. In the head and neck, this procedure can be applied for different nerves, but the most common application is for the medial branch of the primary dorsal ramus, which is the sensory supply of the facet joint in the cervical spine. In addition, this technique has been applied to various nervous structures, including the occipital nerve, with various success rates.

REFERENCES

1. Schweitzer A, Bahr H. Albert Schweitzer letters 1905–1965. New York: MacMillan Publishing Company; 1992.
2. Gallagher RM. Epidural and intrathecal cancer pain management: prescriptive care for quality of life. Pain Med 2004;5:239–47.
3. Feinstein B, Langton JNK, Jameson RM, et al. Experiments on referred pain from deep somatic tissues. J Bone Joint Surg Am 1954;36A:981–7.
4. Hunter CR, Mayfield FH. Role of the upper cervical roots in the production of pain in the head. Am J Surg 1949;78:743–51.
5. Bogduk N, Marsland A. The cervical zygapophysial joints as a source of neck pain. Spine 1988;13:607–10.
6. Bovim G, Berg R. Cervicogenic headache: anesthetic blockades of cervical nerves (C2-C5) and facet joint (C2-C3). Pain 1992;49:315–20.
7. Ymashita T, Cavanaugh J. Mechanosensitive afferent units in the lumbar facet joint. Surgery 1990;72A:865–70.
8. El-Bohy, Cavanaugh J. Localization of substance P and neurofilament immunoreactive fibers in the lumbar facet joint capsule and supraspinous ligament of rabbit. Brain Res 1988;460:379–82.
9. Ahmed M, Bjurholm A. Sensory and autonomic innervation of the facet joint in the rat lumbar spine. Spine 1993;18:2121–6.
10. Dwyer A, Aprill C, Bogduk N. Cervical zygapophysial joint pain patterns. I. A study in normal volunteers. Spine 1990;15:453–7.
11. Sjaastad O, Fredriksen TA, Pfaffenrath V. Cervicogenic headache: diagnostic criteria. Headache 1990;30:725–6.
12. Headache Classification Subcommittee of the International Headache Society. The international classification of headache disorders. 2nd edition. Cephalalgia 2004;24:1–151.
13. Vecht CJ, Hoff AM, Kansen PJ, et al. Types and causes of pain in cancer of the head and neck. Cancer 1992;70:178–84.
14. Sist T, Miner M, Lema M. Characteristics of postradical neck pain syndrome: a report of 25 cases. J Pain Symptom Manage 1999;18(2):95–102.
15. Villaret D, Weymuller E. Pain caused by cancer of the head and neck. In: Loeser J, Butler S, Chapman R, editors. Bonica's management of pain. Philadelphia: Lippincott Williams & Wilkins; 2001. p. 948–65.
16. Foley KM. The treatment of cancer pain. N Engl J Med 1985;313:84–95.
17. Payne R. Cancer pain: anatomy, physiology, and pharmacology. Cancer 1989; 63(Suppl):2266–74.
18. Roodman GD. Mechanisms of bone metastasis. N Engl J Med 2004;350: 1655–64.
19. Honore P, Luger NM, Sabino MA, et al. Osteoprotegerin blocks bone cancer-induced skeletal destruction, skeletal pain and pain-related neurochemical reorganization of the spinal cord. Nat Med 2000;6:521–8.
20. Elliott K, Foley KM. Neurologic pain syndromes in patients with cancer. Crit Care Clin 1990;6:393–420.
21. Jaeckle KA. Causes and management of headaches in cancer patients. Oncology (Huntingt) 1993;7:27–31.
22. Sidebottom A, Maxwell A. The medical and surgical management of trigeminal neuralgia. J Clin Pharm Ther 1995;20:31–5.

23. Murphy T. Somatic blockade of head and neck. In: Cousins M, Bridenbaugh P, editors. Neural blockade in clinical anesthesia and management of pain. Wickford, RI: Lippincott-Raven; 1998. p. 489–514.

24. New York School of Regional Anesthesia. Available at: http://www.nysora.com/techniques/head_neck.

25. Kohase H, Umino M, Shibaji T, et al. Application of a mandibular nerve block using an indwelling catheter for intractable cancer pain. Acta Anaesthesiol Scand 2004;48(3):382–3.

26. Umino M, Kohase H, Ideguchi S, et al. Long-term pain control in trigeminal neuralgia with local anesthetics using an indwelling catheter in the mandibular nerve. Clin J Pain 2002;18(3):196–9.

27. Cooper M, Watson R. An improved regional anaesthetic technique for peroral endoscopy. Anesthesiology 1975;43:372–4.

28. Funasaka S, Kodera K. Intraoral nerve block for glossopharyngeal neuralgia. Arch Otorhinolaryngol 1977;215(3–4):311–5.

29. Bogduk N, Long D. The anatomy of the so-called "articular nerves" and their relationship to facet denervation in the treatment of low back pain. J Neurosurg 1979;51:172–7.

30. Manning D, Rowlingson J. Back pain and the role of neural blockade. In: Cousins M, Bridenbaugh P, editors. Neural blockade in clinical anesthesia and management of pain. Wickford, RI: Lippincott-Raven; 1998. p. 489–514.

The Role of Vestibular Rehabilitation in the Balance Disorder Patient

Courtney D. Hall, PhD, PT[a,b,]*, L. Clarke Cox, PhD[c]

KEYWORDS

- Vestibular rehabilitation • Peripheral vestibular disorder
- Dizziness • Rehabilitation

Dizziness is among the most prevalent complaints for which people seek medical help and is the number one reason for a physician visit for individuals aged more than 75 years.[1,2] Although dizziness can be caused by many different medical conditions, it is estimated that as many as half of cases are due to vestibular disorders.[2,3] Uncompensated vestibular hypofunction results in postural instability, visual blurring, and subjective complaints of imbalance. These serious problems result in decreased activity level, avoidance or modification of driving with resultant diminished independence, limited social interactions, and increased isolation.[4,5]

Studies have shown that the incidence of falls is greater in persons with vestibular hypofunction when compared with healthy individuals of the same age living in the community.[6,7] The potential consequences of a fall include physical harm and loss of independence as well as social embarrassment. The costs of fall-related injuries in older adults are substantial. In the United States alone, it is estimated that annual direct and indirect costs of fall-related injuries will reach $54.9 billion by the year 2020.[8] The psychologic consequences of falls in younger adults have not been studied; however, among older adults who have fallen, nearly half are fearful of falling again, and up to one quarter restrict activities in an attempt to avoid another fall.[9,10]

Dr. Hall was supported in part by Advanced Research Career Development Award E4465K awarded by the Department of Veterans Affairs, Veterans Health Administration, Office of Research and Development.

[a] Atlanta VAMC, Rehabilitation Research and Development Center (151R), 1670 Clairmont Road, Decatur, GA 30033, USA

[b] Department of Rehabilitation Medicine, Emory University, 1441 Clifton Road, NE, Atlanta, GA 30322, USA

[c] Boston University School of Medicine, J.J. Moakley Building, 830 Harrison Avenue, Suite 1400, Boston, MA 02118, USA

* Corresponding author. Atlanta VAMC, Rehabilitation Research and Development Center (151R), 1670 Clairmont Road, Decatur, GA 30033.
E-mail address: chall7@emory.edu (C.D. Hall).

Otolaryngol Clin N Am 42 (2009) 161–169
doi:10.1016/j.otc.2008.09.006
0030-6665/08/$ – see front matter. Published by Elsevier Inc.

Evidence is beginning to accumulate that the use of vestibular rehabilitation is a critical component in improving postural stability and gaze stability and in decreasing subjective complaints of disequilibrium and oscillopsia (perception of visual blurring) for patients with peripheral vestibular loss.[1,11–13] Although these studies differ in the specific details of vestibular rehabilitation, common elements include vestibular adaptation and substitution exercises, balance and gait activities, and general conditioning. The focus of this article is on the role of vestibular rehabilitation in the remediation of postural and gaze instability in individuals with peripheral vestibular deficits. Although vestibular rehabilitation does not cure the organic disease that produces the balance disorder, it improves mobility, prevents falls, and overall has a positive impact on the quality of life for the patient.

MECHANISMS OF RECOVERY

The goals of vestibular rehabilitation are to reduce subjective symptoms, to improve gaze and postural stability (particularly during head movements), and to return the individual to normal activities, including regular physical activity, driving, and work. Vestibular rehabilitation includes exercises to habituate symptoms such as head movement provoked dizziness, exercises to promote vestibular adaptation and substitution, exercises to improve balance and dynamic postural control, and exercises to improve general conditioning.

Compensation for the loss of vestibular function is a process of recovery, with the desired outcome being a return to normal function. Compensation occurs in response to permanent vestibular damage and not to fluctuations in function, such as occurs during the episodic spells of Meniere's disease.

Habituation

One mechanism of compensation is habituation. Habituation refers to the long lasting attenuation of a response to a provocative stimulus brought about by repeated exposure to the provocative stimulus.[14] Habituation exercises are chosen based on particular movements that provoke symptoms in the individual. The Motion Sensitivity Quotient is a standardized assessment in which the patient rates the intensity and duration of dizziness following each of a series of 16 position changes.[15] Habituation as a treatment approach involves systematically provoking symptoms by having the individual perform several repetitions of two to three of the movements or position changes that caused mild-to-moderate symptoms. This systematic repetition of provocative movements leads to a reduction in symptoms. This treatment approach was found to be effective in reducing disability in a group of patients with peripheral and central vestibular deficits. Overall, 82% of the patients reported an improvement in symptoms. Among those with peripheral vestibular deficits, 90% achieved successful outcomes defined as having symptoms that minimally interfered with activities at discharge from rehabilitation. This approach was less successful in individuals with central vestibular disorders as a result of head injury and least successful in individuals with bilateral vestibular hypofunction. For that reason, habituation exercises are not advocated in the treatment of bilateral vestibular loss.[16]

Adaptation

A second mechanism of recovery is adaptation. Adaptation refers to the potential for the remaining vestibular system to adjust its output according to the demands placed on it. Adaptation refers to long-term change in the neuronal response with the goal of reducing symptoms and normalizing gaze and postural stability. A critical signal to induce adaptation is retinal slip during head movements.[17,18] The adaptation exercises involve head movement while maintaining focus on a target which may be stationary or moving (**Fig. 1**). Typical progression of adaptation exercises involves increased velocity of head movement, movement of the target and head, target placement in a distracting visual pattern, and maintenance of a challenging posture. **Table 1** presents a sample progression of vestibular adaptation and substitution exercises. Adaptation exercises alone have been found to reduce symptoms of disequilibrium and to improve balance while walking in individuals who are post surgery for resection of acoustic neuroma.[11]

Substitution

A third mechanism of recovery is substitution. The goal is to substitute alternative strategies for missing vestibular function. Potential substitution for the vestibulo-ocular reflex (VOR) includes the cervical ocular reflex, use of smooth pursuit eye movements, and central preprogramming of eye movements. Substitution for the vestibulospinal reflex includes the use of visual, somatosensory cues, or both to maintain stability.[1,19,20] Substitution exercises specifically attempt to facilitate the use of alternative strategies rather than teaching the specific strategies. For example, during a remembered target exercise, the individual attempts to maintain eye position on a target with the eyes closed, potentially facilitating use of the cervical ocular reflex. During active eye-head exercise, a large eye movement to a target is made before the head moving to face the target, potentially facilitating the use of preprogrammed eye movements.

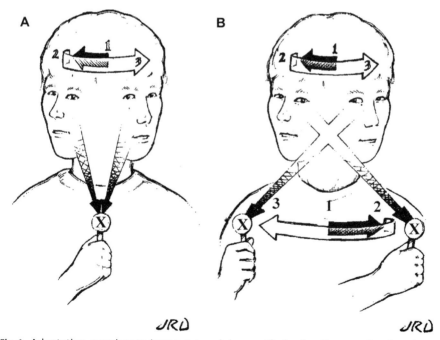

Fig. 1. Adaptation exercises to improve remaining vestibular function require that the patient attempt to fixate on a visual target (either stationary, *A*, or moving, *B*) during either horizontal or vertical head movement. Exercises in which the target is stationary are referred to as VOR X1 and those in which the target is moving as VOR X2. (*From* Tusa RJ, Herdman SJ. Vertigo and disequilibrium. In: Johnson R, Griffith J, editors. Current therapy in neurologic disease. Edition 4. St. Louis: Mosby Year-Book; 1993. p. 12; with permission.)

Table 1
Sample progression of exercises

Time Period	Exercise	Duration	Frequency	Total Time[a]
Week 1	X1 viewing, foveal target, distant, horizontal/vertical	1 min	5×/d	20
	X1 viewing, foveal target, near, horizontal/vertical	1 min	5×/d	
Week 2	X1 viewing, foveal target, distant, horizontal/vertical	1 min	5×/d	40
	X1 viewing, foveal target, near, horizontal/vertical	1 min	5×/d	
	Active eye-head, near, horizontal/vertical	2 min	5×/d	
Week 3	X1 viewing, foveal target, distant, horizontal/vertical	1.5 min	5×/d	50
	X1 viewing, foveal target, near, horizontal/vertical	1.5 min	5×/d	
	X1 viewing paradigm, full-field target, near, horizontal	1 min	5×/d	
	Active eye-head, near, horizontal/vertical	2 min	3×/d	
	Remembered targets, near, horizontal	1 min	3×/d	
Week 4	X1 viewing paradigm, full-field target, near, horizontal/vertical	1 min	4×/d	40
	X2 viewing paradigm, foveal target, near, horizontal/vertical	1 min	4×/d	
	Active eye-head, near, horizontal/vertical	2 min	2×/d	
	Remembered targets, near, horizontal/vertical	2 min	2×/d	
	Walk with head turns, horizontal/vertical	2-3 min	2×/d	
Week 5	X1 viewing, foveal target, near, horizontal/vertical	1 min	4×/d	40
	X1 viewing paradigm, full-field target, near, horizontal/vertical	1 min	4×/d	
	X2 viewing paradigm, foveal target, near, horizontal/vertical	1 min	2×/d	
	Active eye-head, distant, horizontal/vertical	1 min	2×/d	
	Remembered targets, near, horizontal/vertical	1 min	2×/d	
Week 6	X1 viewing paradigm, full-field target, near, horizontal/vertical	1 min	5×/d	55
	X2 viewing paradigm, foveal target, near, horizontal/vertical	1.5 min	5×/d	
	Active eye-head, distant, horizontal/vertical	1 min	5×/d	
	Remembered targets, near, horizontal/vertical	1 min	5×/d	
	Walk with head turns, horizontal/vertical, cognitive task	5 min	5×/d	

[a] Time in minutes plus walking as an exercise.

From Hall CD, Herdman SJ. Balance, vestibular and oculomotor dysfunction. In: Selzer ME, Cohen L, Gage FH, et al, editors. Textbook of neural repair and rehabilitation. Cambridge (UK): Cambridge University Press; 2006. p. 298–314.

In addition to exercises specifically geared to the vestibular system, balance exercises under challenging sensory and dynamic conditions are typically included as part of vestibular rehabilitation. Static exercises include balancing under conditions of altered visual and somatosensory input. The tasks are made more challenging by progressively narrowing the base of support. Dynamic conditions challenge high level balance and include walking with head turns, walking with quick turns to the right or left, or performing a secondary task while walking such as tossing a ball to a partner or performing a cognitive task while walking.

Many individuals with vestibular hypofunction limit regular physical activities. Although general conditioning alone does not reduce symptoms or improve postural stability,[1] including physical activity is an important element of rehabilitation. The authors recommend that every patient start a progressive walking program, ideally outside, and increase to 20 to 30 minutes on a daily basis.

THE ROLE OF VESTIBULAR REHABILITATION IN RECOVERY OF FUNCTION

Several randomized controlled studies support the conclusion that vestibular exercises are important in the rehabilitation of patients with vestibular disorders.[1,11–13] These studies are important because they provide the first evidence that vestibular exercises result in improved function when compared with a control group. Vestibular rehabilitation accelerates recovery of postural stability and subjective symptoms of disequilibrium following acute vestibular loss.[11,21] In these studies, vestibular rehabilitation was started within 3 days following surgical resection of acoustic neuroma. The vestibular rehabilitation group reported significantly fewer subjective symptoms and displayed significantly fewer gait deviations than the control group at the time of discharge.

Vestibular Exercise

General effects
There does not seem to be a critical period during which vestibular exercises must be started to see improvement; however, starting rehabilitation sooner has the important effect of reducing fall risk and potentially reducing fall incidence. Vestibular rehabilitation has been found to be beneficial even in individuals with chronic dizziness.[1,13,14,22,23] Horak and colleagues[1] found that 6 weeks of vestibular rehabilitation led to significant improvements in postural control and symptoms, whereas medication (meclizine) or general exercise only reduced symptoms. Szturm and colleagues[23] compared a home program of standard vestibular habituation exercises versus customized vestibular rehabilitation. The customized vestibular rehabilitation group demonstrated significant improvement in postural stability, whereas the home exercise group did not change. In addition, VOR asymmetry was improved for the customized vestibular rehabilitation group but not for the home exercise group. When compared with standard medical care, vestibular rehabilitation was found to improve symptoms of anxiety and depression, disability, motion sensitivity, and performance on tests of static balance.[13] Individuals with unilateral or bilateral vestibular hypofunction make significant gains with vestibular rehabilitation; however, individuals with bilateral vestibular hypofunction improve to a lesser extent.[12]

Effect on gaze stability
The role of vestibular exercises in the recovery of gaze stability during head movement (dynamic visual acuity) has received little attention to date. Without the VOR, gaze stabilization during head movement is poor; therefore, visual cues to help maintain postural stability would not be particularly useful. Even at a static visual acuity of 20/40,

postural stability is reduced. Two recent studies demonstrated that vestibular rehabilitation improved dynamic visual acuity in patients with peripheral (unilateral and bilateral) vestibular hypofunction.[24,25] As a group, patients who performed vestibular exercises showed a significant improvement in visual acuity during head movement (as measured with computerized testing), whereas those performing placebo exercises did not (**Fig. 2**). Statistical analysis revealed that the leading factor contributing to the improvement was vestibular exercise. Other factors such as age, the time from onset, and subjective symptoms did not affect the outcome of rehabilitation.

Effect on fall risk

Little research has examined the role of vestibular rehabilitation in reducing fall risk. In a retrospective study of patients with bilateral vestibular hypofunction, vestibular rehabilitation resulted in a limited reduction in fall risk as measured by the Dynamic Gait Index score.[26] Following vestibular rehabilitation, patients improved in several outcome measures (including balance-related confidence and disability), but the majority of those initially at risk for falls were still at risk at discharge. In contrast, a retrospective study of individuals with unilateral vestibular hypofunction found that vestibular rehabilitation resulted in a significant reduction in fall risk.[27] In that study, the majority of subjects (68%) were at low risk for falls at discharge (**Fig. 3**). The difference in results between these two studies suggests that the degree of vestibular loss influences outcomes. Individuals with bilateral vestibular loss will likely continue to be at risk for falls, whereas individuals with unilateral loss will likely be at low risk for falls at discharge from therapy.

Vestibular Rehabilitation

Group versus individual findings

Typically, published reports on the efficacy of vestibular rehabilitation do not provide information at the individual level. For example, the number of subjects within a group (treatment or control) who do not show improvement is typically not reported. With few exceptions, the studies reported in this article did not examine the effect of specific factors such as exercise approach, gender, the time from onset, psychologic factors, comorbidities, or the environment on the recovery of function. Relatively few studies of patients with vestibular hypofunction clearly state that some patients do not improve.

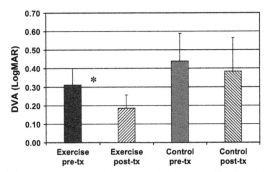

Fig. 2. There is significant improvement in dynamic visual acuity for patients with bilateral vestibular hypofunction who receive vestibular exercise but not placebo exercise. Data are reported as mean +1 SD. LogMAR = logarithm of the minimal angle of resolution. (*P = .001). (*From* Herdman SJ, Hall CD, Schubert MC, et al. Recovery of dynamic visual acuity in bilateral vestibular hypofunction. Arch Otolaryngol Head Neck Surg 2007;133:387; with permission.)

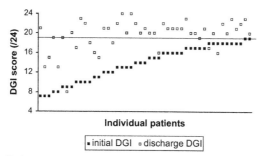

Fig. 3. Initial and discharge Dynamic Gait Index (DGI) scores are plotted for individual patients with unilateral vestibular hypofunction. The line is positioned at a DGI score of 19/24, with scores at or below considered at risk for falls. Scores falling above the line indicate patients who are at low risk for falls. (*From* Hall CD, Schubert MC, Herdman SJ. Prediction of fall risk reduction as measured by Dynamic Gait Index in individuals with unilateral vestibular hypofunction. Otol Neurotol 2004;25:748; with permission.)

Of patients with unilateral vestibular hypofunction, depending upon which outcome measure is used, between 10% and 30% of subjects do not improve.[27–29] Of patients with bilateral vestibular hypofunction, outcomes are worse, with 25% to 66% of patients failing to show improvement.[24,26,28] These findings are extremely important because, as clinicians, we deal with individuals and not groups.

Implementation into clinical practice
Questions remain regarding specific recommendations for implementation of vestibular rehabilitation into clinical practice. Little is known about whether all exercise approaches are uniformly beneficial for different types of vestibular hypofunction. Although one group found that habituation was not effective in the treatment of bilateral vestibular hypofunction,[16] no studies have compared the relative effectiveness of different exercise approaches (habituation, adaptation, substitution) directly. An additional confound is the issue of supervision. Certain studies examined the benefits of different treatment approaches but also used different levels of supervision. For example, Szturm[23] compared a supervised exercise program with a home exercise program, but the supervised exercises were based on adaptation and the home exercise program was based on habituation. Another obstacle to identifying the most appropriate treatment approach is the tremendous variety from study to study in terms of the number and frequency of clinic visits as well as the intensity of the home exercise program. Visits to the clinic varied from several times a week to once a week to a single follow-up telephone call after initial evaluation. The prescribed frequency of performance of the exercises at home has been reported to be as few as twice a day up to five times a day. Much work remains to be done to determine appropriate practice patterns, because different studies have used different exercise approaches, different outcome measures, and different patient populations.

SUMMARY

Despite the questions that remain regarding the specific details of vestibular rehabilitation, there is no doubt that vestibular rehabilitation contributes significantly to the successful treatment of peripheral vestibular disorders. Prospective controlled studies have provided evidence that vestibular rehabilitation is beneficial in improving postural and gaze stability as well as decreasing subjective complaints for patients with vestibular hypofunction. The age of the patient, the time from onset, and the severity of symptoms do not prevent significant improvement in outcomes following vestibular rehabilitation. Although not all patients achieve normal function, it is expected that the majority of patients will achieve normal postural and gaze stability with head movements and will report only minimal subjective symptoms. Vestibular rehabilitation allows for most patients with peripheral vestibular hypofunction to return to normal activities of daily living and a high quality of life.

REFERENCES

1. Horak FB, Jones-Rycewicz C, Black FO, et al. Effects of vestibular rehabilitation on dizziness and imbalance. Otolaryngol Head Neck Surg 1992;106:175–80.
2. Kroenke K, Lucas CA, Rosenberg ML, et al. Causes of persistent dizziness: a prospective study of 100 patients in ambulatory care. Ann Intern Med 1992;117: 898–904.
3. Cohen HS, Kimball KT. Development of the vestibular disorders activities of daily living scale. Arch Otolaryngol Head Neck Surg 2000;126:881–7.
4. Cohen HS, Wells J, Kimball KT, et al. Driving disability and dizziness. J Safety Res 2003;34:361–9.
5. Yardley L, Verschuur C, Masson E, et al. Somatic and psychological factors contributing to handicap in people with vertigo. Br J Audiol 1992;26:283–90.
6. Herdman SJ, Blatt P, Schubert MC, et al. Falls in patients with vestibular deficits. Am J Otol 2000;21:847–51.
7. Pothula VB, Chew F, Lesser THJ, et al. Falls and vestibular impairment. Clin Otolaryngol 2004;29:179–82.
8. National Center for Injury Prevention and Control. Costs of falls among older adults. Available at: http://www.cdc.gov/ncipc/factsheets/fallcost.htm. Accessed October 15, 2008.
9. Murphy SL, Williams CS, Gill TM. Characteristics associated with fear of falling and activity restriction in community-living older persons. J Am Geriatr Soc 2002;50:516–20.
10. Yardley L, Smith H. A prospective study of the relationship between feared consequences of falling and avoidance of activity in community-living older people. Gerontologist 2002;42:17–23.
11. Herdman SJ, Clendaniel RA, Mattox DE, et al. Vestibular adaptation exercises and recovery: acute stage after acoustic neuroma resection. Otolaryngol Head Neck Surg 1995;113:77–87.
12. Krebs DE, Gill-Body KM, Riley PO, et al. Double-blind, placebo-controlled trial of rehabilitation for bilateral vestibular hypofunction: preliminary report. Otolaryngol Head Neck Surg 1993;109:735–41.
13. Yardley L, Beech S, Zander L, et al. A randomized controlled trial of exercise therapy for dizziness and vertigo in primary care. Br J Gen Pract 1998;48: 1136–40.
14. Telian SA, Shepard NT, Smith-Wheelock M, et al. Habituation therapy for chronic vestibular dysfunction: preliminary results. Otolaryngol Head Neck Surg 1990; 103:89–95.
15. Smith-Wheelock M, Shepard NT, Telian SA. Physical therapy program for vestibular rehabilitation. Am J Otol 1991;12:218–25.
16. Telian SA, Shepard NT, Smith-Wheelock M, et al. Bilateral vestibular paresis: diagnosis and treatment. Otolaryngol Head Neck Surg 1991;104:67–71.
17. Gauthier GM, Robinson DA. Adaptation of the human vestibulo-ocular reflex to magnifying lenses. Brain Res 1975;92:331–5.

18. Shelhamer M, Tiliket C, Roberts D, et al. Short-term vestibulo-ocular reflex adaptation in humans. II. Error signals. Exp Brain Res 1994;100:328–36.
19. Herdman SJ, Schubert MC, Tusa RJ. Role of central preprogramming in dynamic visual acuity with vestibular loss. Arch Otolaryngol Head Neck Surg 2001;127: 1205–10.
20. Schubert MC, Das V, Tusa RJ, et al. Cervico-ocular reflex in normal subjects and patients with unilateral vestibular hypofunction. Otol Neurotol 2004;25: 65–71.
21. Enticott JC, O'Leary SJ, Briggs RJ. Effects of vestibulo-ocular reflex exercises on vestibular compensation after vestibular Schwannoma surgery. Otol Neurotol 2005;26:265–9.
22. Black FO, Angel CR, Pesznecker SC, et al. Outcome analysis of individualized vestibular rehabilitation protocols. Am J Otol 2000;21:543–51.
23. Szturm T, Ireland DJ, Lessing-Turner M. Comparison of different exercise programs in the rehabilitation of patients with chronic peripheral vestibular dysfunction. J Vestib Res 1994;4:461–79.
24. Herdman SJ, Hall CD, Schubert MC, et al. Recovery of dynamic visual acuity in bilateral vestibular hypofunction. Arch Otolaryngol Head Neck Surg 2007;133: 383–9.
25. Herdman SJ, Schubert MC, Das VE, et al. Recovery of dynamic visual acuity in unilateral vestibular hypofunction. Arch Otolaryngol Head Neck Surg 2003;129: 819–24.
26. Brown KE, Whitney SL, Wrisley DM, et al. Physical therapy outcomes for persons with bilateral vestibular loss. Laryngoscope 2001;111:1812–7.
27. Hall CD, Schubert MC, Herdman SJ. Prediction of fall risk reduction as measured by Dynamic Gait Index in individuals with unilateral vestibular hypofunction. Otol Neurotol 2004;25:746–51.
28. Krebs DE, Gill-Body KM, Parker SW, et al. Vestibular rehabilitation: useful but not universally so. Otolaryngol Head Neck Surg 2003;128:240–50.
29. Topuz O, Topuz B, Ardiç FN, et al. Efficacy of vestibular rehabilitation on chronic unilateral vestibular dysfunction. Clin Rehabil 2004;18:76–83.

Living with Head and Neck Cancer and Coping with Dying when Treatments Fail

Alphi Elackattu, MD, Scharukh Jalisi, MD*

KEYWORDS

• Palliative • Cancer • Death • Dying

It has been suggested that many cancer patients die an undignified death with poorly controlled symptoms.[1] A good death is one that is pain free, peaceful, and dignified, at a place of choosing with the relatives present and without futile heroic interventions.[2] Although the notion of dying at home may be a romantic ideal among health care professionals who aim to provide a good death, as symptoms accelerate in the last 24 to 48 hours, some patients and their families may feel overwhelmed by concerns about symptom control or a dead body at home and therefore prefer a skilled care environment.[3] Previous quality of care studies have identified effective pain and symptom management as the overwhelming priority for patients and their caregivers, closely followed by preservation of the patients' dignity and hygiene.[4] In a meta-analysis of 52 studies, den Beuken and colleagues[5] found the pooled prevalence of pain to be greater than 50% in all cancer types, with the highest prevalence in patients who had head and neck cancer (70%; 95% CI, 51% to 88%).

In their study, Fried and colleagues[3] provide good insight into the final moments of a patient's end of life. Pain was a common symptom (84%) and was managed successfully in all patients, with 93% receiving opioids. Management of other symptoms, except neuropsychologic problems, was satisfactory. Sixty-three percent of patients died in the hospital, and only 22% had a relative present at the time of death. Resuscitation status was documented in only 65% of the notes, although none of the patients were admitted to the ICU or underwent resuscitation. Fifty-three percent of patients were admitted as an emergency in the last month of life, and bleeding was the most common cause of admission.

Department of Otolaryngology-Head and Neck Surgery, Boston University Medical Center, Boston, MA, USA
* Corresponding author. Department of Otolaryngology—Head and Neck Surgery, Boston University Medical Center, Boston, MA.
E-mail address: scharukh.jalisi@bmc.org (S. Jalisi).

Otolaryngol Clin N Am 42 (2009) 171–184
doi:10.1016/j.otc.2008.09.004
0030-6665/08/$ – see front matter © 2009 Elsevier Inc. All rights reserved.

TALKING TO THE FAMILY
When Cure is not Possible

Some criteria of when to forgo treatment for advanced cancer are based on poor performance status, age greater than 70 years (for chemotherapy), the previous treatment performed (prior doses of radiation and chemotherapy), the extent of cancer, and expected survival.[6] Widely metastatic disease, including lung and bone metastases, is incurable. Subjecting such a patient to a complex surgery can be a setback in their quality of life without achieving any benefit from a survival standpoint. The patient's overall health status is important. If they have poor cardiopulmonary function, surgery itself may result in death or stroke. Age is no longer a limitation to providing care in the authors' practice because the aging population is resulting in healthier octogenarians who can withstand the rigors of cancer therapy. Moreover, prior radiotherapy may preclude additional radiotherapy due to the risk of inducing further cancer. Our treatment paradigm is to preserve the quality of life of individuals to the best possible extent and to carefully weigh the risks and benefits of any therapy (surgical or nonsurgical) against the wishes of the patient and family.

Breaking the News to the Family

Honest and open communication is of utmost importance during the sensitive and life-altering moments people face when confronted with cancer that may ultimately be fatal. Hallenbeck and colleagues[7] noted some key points that should be addressed whenever dealing with such a situation. They stress that, during this confusing time, it is important to ensure that the patient and their family understand the diagnosis and prognosis. Because the treatment has moved from cure to palliation, new goals must be set. As palliative care progresses, the health care team and the family must constantly reassess new symptoms that may occur with changing treatments. Physicians should be willing to discuss the treatment options and be willing to make recommendations. Even in the most dire situations, there is always something that can be done for the patient, such as a change in pain medication or an exercise routine. Most importantly, one must never abandon a patient in this greatest time of need.

Cultural sensitivity must be taken into account. In several cultures, including those from South Asia, the diagnosis of cancer itself is a death sentence. In such a situation family involvement is an excellent intermediary to help the patient achieve the best treatment and have realistic goals.

In the authors' practice, a team approach is used to understand the concerns of the patient and family. Sometimes the patient may not be willing to discuss something that they consider inconsequential for the physician but are comfortable discussing with a nurse or medical assistant. At a minimum, a successful head and neck cancer practice must have a cancer nurse, a cancer nurse practitioner, and a cancer patient navigator available. This staffing provides for several layers of social support, medical support, and guidance for the many tests or appointments a patient may have to deal with. Such a service greatly enhances patient and family satisfaction with the care they receive.

PALLIATIVE MEASURES
Chemoradiation Therapy

The decision of when to pursue curative versus palliative treatment with chemoradiation is often a difficult choice and requires open communication with the patient and family. When the decision is made for palliative treatment, the goal must be to provide optimal relief while minimizing the side effects of treatment and remembering that cure is not the goal. A study by Graf and colleagues[8] sought to determine whether treating with concomitant radiation and chemotherapy would be superior to the traditional method of sequential treatment with induction chemotherapy followed by radiation in inoperable head and neck cancers. The sequential protocol started with two courses of neoadjuvant chemotherapy, cisplatin and 5-fluorouracil, followed by a course of radiotherapy using conventional fractionation up to 70 Gy. The concomitant protocol used two courses of 5-fluorouracil plus mitomycin along with a course of radiotherapy up to 30 Gy in conventional fractionation, which was followed by a hyperfractionated course up to 72 Gy. There were significant increases in response rate and local control along with a trend toward higher disease-specific and overall survival rates after 5 years in the group that received concomitant radiation and chemotherapy followed by radiation. Late toxicity was found to be similar in both groups. A study by Yogi and Singh[9] of 100 patients showed improved survival and symptom relief when induction therapy was used before combined chemoradiotherapy as opposed to induction chemotherapy and radiation. In a study by Mohanti and colleagues,[10] 505 patients with nonmetastatic stage IV head and neck cancer received 20 Gy in five fractions over 1 week, along with medication for symptom relief. Symptom relief was achieved for greater than 50% of the patients. The following responses rates were observed: relief of pain, 57%; dysphagia, 53%; hoarseness, 57%; cough, 59%; and otalgia, 47%. The overall survival ranged from 34 to 2065 days. Teymoortash and colleagues[11] performed a study in which they intra-arterially injected cisplatin into unresectable head and neck tumors. They reported a decrease in malodor, pain, and tumor bleeding. This method may be an approach to consider when palliatively treating such patients.

Debulking

The major morbidity from advanced head and neck cancer is airway obstruction, dysphagia, pain, and bleeding. Forbes[12] stated that the goal of palliative surgery is to improve the patient's quality of life by reducing symptoms without the additive effect of surgical complications. He made several observations concerning the role of surgery in palliation and the principles of preoperative care, operation for advanced cancer, and postoperative care (**Box 1**).

Cancer of the head and neck often necessitates adjunctive treatments to provide patients with adequate voice use or to allow them to swallow. Tumor debulking can be a useful adjunct to palliation or can prepare patients for chemotherapy, radiotherapy, or definite surgery. There are many advantages to the laser as a debulking agent. It is quick, repeatable, and coagulates tissue, and it is atraumatic, precise, and allows for sterilization and prompt healing.[13] Laccourreye and colleagues[14] in a 10-year study of 42 patients used the CO_2 laser to debulk endolaryngeal cancers. They were able to achieve a 95% success rate in patients awaiting definitive treatment for their disease and an 87.5% success rate in patients who were undergoing palliation. Recently, Phelan and colleagues[15] reported successful debulking with the use of microdebriders to reestablish airways in patients with obstructing laryngeal tumors. Paleri and colleagues[16] reviewed the records of 50 patients who underwent laser debulking for airway obstruction that was caused by laryngeal or hypopharyngeal malignancies, with 14 of these patients only receiving palliative measures. For their patient population, the mean number of procedures was 1.9, with 1% to 6.91% of patients avoiding a tracheostomy. The avoidance of tracheostomy in these patients is of great benefit, because there has been a reported risk of 8% to 41%[17] for tumor seeding of the peristomal wound with resultant recurrence after laryngectomy.

Box 1
Forbes' observations concerning the goals of palliative surgery

The role of surgery in palliation

1. Cancer patients are surgical patients first.
2. Surgery is directed at the consequences of the tumor.
3. Integrate surgery into specific treatment and supportive care.
4. Avoid unreasonable delay of palliative surgery.
5. Surgical problems may have a benign cause; obtain histology.

Principles of preoperative care

1. Perform consultations and provide explanations.
2. Plan for immediate and long-term care.

Principles of operating for advanced cancer

1. Determine the site of incision.
2. Each patient must undergo the procedure that is optimal for him or her.

Principles of postoperative care

1. Optimize recovery by avoiding complications.
2. Obtain an early diagnosis and perform aggressive management of complications.

Tumor debulking provides an avenue to improve the airway and possibly avoid a tracheotomy, to reduce pain by reducing tumor bulk, to reduce the chance of a major bleed, and to possibly remove an anatomic hindrance to successful swallowing (although most patients at this stage have had surgery or chemoradiation or both that have effected swallowing at baseline). Tumor debulking has the potential to improve the overall quality of life in this patient population.

Managing the External Fungating Lesion

Patients often suffer great psychosocial and physical distress due to the unremitting and debilitating process of a fungating lesion. Patients may see their bodies morphologically changed, affecting their confidence and willingness to interact socially. Additionally, they often exude a malodor that impacts their interactions. Grocott[18] has suggested three tools to aid in malodor: systemic antibiotics, topical metronidazole, and charcoal dressings.

The care of wounds is often a complicated process. When possible, a consultation with wound care teams must be immediately sought. Only wounds that are producing excessive exudates, purulence, or serous fluids require cleansing.[19] This cleansing can be adequately done with showering, but a sterile technique must be used if there is deep bone involvement. Dressings should be able to maintain moisture to avoid adherence to the wound and at the same time be able to vent excess fluid. Debridement of necrotic tissue may provide the benefits of reducing infection, exudates, and malodor. Because sharp debridement carries the risk of hemorrhage, for most patients the debridement provided by moist dressings will be adequate. Nutritional support should be provided if high amounts of exudates are noted, because exudates are protein rich. Pain control from the tumor should be frequently assessed and treated. Proper and early referrals should be made to the appropriate team members.

COMPLICATIONS FROM PALLIATIVE MEASURES
The Effects of Altered Anatomy

Our physical appearance places a large role in our everyday life and is often taken for granted. It is important for self-confidence, our interactions with people, and our ability to effectively communicate. Patients suffer greatly when their physical appearance becomes altered in the course of surgical treatment. No two patients have the same scars, heal the same, or have the same perceptions about their appearance. Two studies have made some strong points on this topic.

Rumsey and colleagues[20] studied 220 outpatients who were receiving treatment for burns, skin conditions, or head and neck cancer, or seeking plastic surgery for other appearance concerns. The study revealed that these patients displayed raised levels of anxiety, depression, social anxiety, social avoidance, and a reduced quality of life. Levels of psychosocial distress were not well correlated with the severity of disfigurement; therefore, individual assessment is crucial. Katz and colleagues[21] studied 82 ambulatory head and neck cancer patients who were assessed at least 6 months after treatment and disease free. They found a discrepancy between the way men and women felt about the changes to their body. On the Atkinson Life Happiness Rating scale, the mean was 7.78 (standard deviation [SD], 1.93) on a scale from 1 to 11, which indicates an overall satisfaction with life. Men reported a significantly higher mean life happiness (8.11; SD, 2.01) when compared with women (7.04; SD, 1.54), (t [80] = 2.36, $P<.02$). The researchers also reported increased depressive symptoms for women and for those who were more disfigured. Social support was not related to depressive symptom levels.

In the authors' surgical practice, the early recognition of these symptoms is key via a multidisciplinary approach and multiple tiers of care providers. We provide early referral to psychology and have established a head and neck cancer support group to help patients and their families cope with the situation.

Speech in the Alaryngeal Patient

The reader is referred to the article by Grillone and Langmore, elsewhere in this issue for more information on this topic.

Swallowing

The reader is referred to the article by Kozak and Grundfast, elsewhere in this issue for more information on this topic.

Exposed Carotid Artery in a Radiated Field

The presence of an exposed carotid artery in the radiated field is a challenging situation with a high morbidity and mortality. Such patients are at risk of carotid blowout with resultant exsanguination. The patient needs to be transferred to an ICU setting for close neurovascular checks. The patient with such a condition should be clearly explained the risks ahead, and an understanding and documentation of their code status is essential. If the patient is full code, an emergent coverage of the defect with a muscle flap is essential. The pectoralis major myocutaneous flap or lower island trapezius muscle flap are good choices for thick muscle coverage for the carotid artery. During the time that the patient is waiting for surgery, the carotid needs to be kept wet with normal saline wet-to-wet dressing changes. If the patient has a do not resuscitate order or declines surgery, palliative saline dressing changes are needed with the understanding that they will be associated with carotid blowout and resultant death.

Role of Regional or Microvascular Free Tissue Transplant Reconstruction in the Nonhealing Tissue Bed

Major reconstruction of treatment-related defects is often part of head and neck cancer care. Reconstruction is often complicated by concomitant treatments such as radiation. The risk of complications in a primarily radiated field can be as high as 30%. Sandel and Davidson[22] reviewed the records of 14 patients who had 16 free flaps to assess the success of free flaps for radiation-induced damage which did not heal after 3 months. Twelve patients had osteoradionecrosis, nine had mandible involvement, and three had scalp involvement. Osteoradionecrosis can be a devastating late consequence of radiation that can be hard to treat, with morbidity ranging from pain, infection, and fistula formation to dysphagia. Free tissue transplants had a good healing rate in a radiated bed. There was a slightly higher rate of skin paddle breakdown and fistula formation in the radionecrosis group. The findings suggested that, overall, advanced stage III radionecrosis of the bone or soft tissue does just as well with free tissue transplant reconstruction as other diseases, and vascular anastomosis may be more successful if performed outside the radiated field, although the patient numbers were not large enough to statistically prove this.

Mucositis in the Patient Undergoing Radiotherapy

Oral mucositis is a painful inflammatory process characterized by ulcers on oral mucosa covered by a pseudomembrane and is a common consequence of radiation and chemotherapy. Oral mucositis results from two major mechanisms: direct toxicity to the oral mucosa and myelosuppression due to the treatment. Its pathophysiology is composed of four interdependent phases: an initial inflammatory/vascular phase, an epithelial phase, an ulcerative/bacteriologic phase, and a healing phase. It is considered a potential source of life-threatening infection and often is a dose-limiting factor in anticancer therapy.[23] Breaks in treatment that are often caused by this complication can lead to tumor repopulation and have negative effects on chemo- and radiotherapy. Patients with oral mucositis are significantly more likely to have severe pain and a weight loss of greater than 5% when compared with similar patients and require $1700 to $6000 more for treatment.[24] Currently, the care of patients with mucositis is essentially palliative, relying on oral hygiene, a nonirritating diet, and oral care products including topical mouth rinses, anesthetics, and the use of systemic opioid analgesics.

Aziz and Ebenfelt[25] in a study of 10 patients discovered that 8 of the patients had increased numbers of granulocytes without macrophage activity in their secretions after 2 weeks of radiotherapy. All of these patients developed mucositis. They suggested that the granulocytes in the secretion may have a role in the development of mucositis during radiotherapy. This connection is supported by a study by Patnie and colleagues[26] who observed a decreased severity of mucositis and dysphagia in patients treated with granulocyte macrophage-colony stimulating factor. Other treatment options include amifostine, which has been found to reduce the severity of acute mucositis and acute and late xerostomia in patients who have head and neck cancer.[27] Initial reports of the use of the immunokine WF10 suggest that it appears to reduce the severity of oropharyngeal complications such as mucositis and dysphagia associated with standard radiation and chemotherapy.[28]

Xerostomia

Xerostomia is a subjective feeling of dry mouth, usually due to a decrease in saliva production. It is often a permanent complication of head and neck cancer treatment with radiotherapy and chemotherapy. It occurs in nearly all patients undergoing radio-therapy and directly affects quality of life in the long run. Saliva has many important roles that are often taken for granted, such as aiding in speech and swallowing and providing antimicrobial protection. In a study of 16 patients with advanced malignan-cies, symptomatic xerostomia, and its associated symptoms, the condition had a considerable negative global impact, resulting in shame, anxiety, disappointments, and verbal communication difficulties.[29]

Jellema and colleagues[30] evaluated patients with stage I to IV disease without distant metastases and found a significant association of radiation-induced xerosto-mia and overall quality of life. In terms of gender, this process had a greater impact on women, and there was a marked worsening of quality of life with increasing xero-stomia. The impact of xerostomia on quality of life increased the longer the patient sustained the disease. In addition to the discomfort, these patients are also more prone to oral diseases such as candidiasis.[31]

Treatment consists of three pathways: (1) increasing saliva production by mechan-ical (eg, chewing gum), gustatory (eg, vitamin C tablets), or pharmacologic stimulation (eg, pilocarpine); (2) using saliva substitutes; and (3) improving active mouth care. A soft diet must be advised; hard and dry food, tobacco, and alcoholic beverages should be avoided.[32] A new treatment modality that has shown promising results is transcutaneous electric nerve stimulation. This new modality has been successful in increasing parotid gland salivary flow in two thirds of healthy adult subjects.[33]

Prevention is better than cure, and some promising new options can be considered before treatment of this patient population. Data in a rat model suggest that pretreat-ment with cevimeline, a muscarinic receptor agonist, prevents radiation-induced xerostomia and the radiation-induced decrease in expression of AQP5 in submandib-ular glands.[34] A potential surgical option is the Seikaly-Jha procedure, which is a method of preserving a single submandibular gland by surgically transferring it to the submental space before radiotherapy. Improved radiation techniques such as intensity-modulated radiotherapy and tomotherapy allow more selective delivery of radiation to defined targets in the head and neck, preserving normal tissue and the salivary glands.[35]

MECHANISMS OF DEATH
Natural Course of Head and Neck Cancer

It is important to be familiar with the natural course of disease and how patients suc-cumb to their illness in lieu of treatment when making the choice as to what, if any, treatment should be undertaken. Many factors must be taken into account, such as the stage of the disease, the survival rates, associated morbidities with treatment, and the natural course of the specific disease entity. Kowalski and Carvalho[6] reviewed 808 untreated head and neck cancer cases that were given only supportive care due to advanced tumor stage, poor performance states, or the patients' refusal of any treatment. Ninety-seven percent of the patients were at clinically advanced stage III or IV. Patients were receiving supportive measures including pain medications and ad-ditionally tracheotomy (6.7%), enteral nutrition (1.6%), and gastrostomy (1.5%). The overall survival of patients ranged from 1 day to 53.8 months (mean, 3.82 months), with about 50% of untreated patients dying within 4 months of their diagnosis. The age, gender, race, and length of time from symptoms to diagnosis did not influence survival; rather, the most significant predictors were clinical stage, tumor site, and per-formance score. The 1- and 3-year survival rates were 27.8% and 1.1% for the larynx, 26.5% and 2.9% for the lip, 15.8% and 0.5% for the oral cavity, 14.4% and 1.7% for the oropharynx, and 12% and 0% for the hypopharynx, respectively. Historically, the definition of "unresectable," which patients should undergo tracheotomy, and other such factors has changed over the 37-year period this review was conducted. The proportion of untreated patients has decreased from 30% in the 1950s to 8.6% in the 1980s; however, the authors did not find any correlation with these changes and survival.

General Causes of Death

Wutzle and colleagues[36] examined the cause of death for patients with cancer of the oral cavity who underwent multimodality treatment. Patients received preoperative radiotherapy of 50 Gy, concomitant chemotherapy with mitomycin and 5-fluorouracil, and radical locoregional en bloc resection. After a median surveillance period of 72.3 months (range, 24 to 152 months), 131 of the 222 patients (41%) had died. Twenty-one percent had died of recurrence, 5% had died perioperatively, and 15% had died of other causes (eg, pneumonia, 6; acute respiratory distress syndrome, 4; stroke, 2; myocardial infarction, 2; asphyxia, 2; heart failure, 1; and chronic obstructive pulmonary disease, 2). Of those who died, a second cancer in the head and neck region, lower respiratory tract, or the upper digestive tract was found in 7.3%. Forty-six (20.7%) died of a recurrent tumor, 9 patients (4%) died because of pulmonary cancer, 4 patients (1.8%) died as the result of a fatal second cancer, 3 patients (1.4%) died because of esophageal cancer, and 2 patients (1%) died of other second cancers. Twelve deaths (5.4%) occurred perioperatively, 15 patients (6.7%) died of internal disease, and 40 patients (18%) had at least one major disease in addition to the immediate cause of death; however, the additional disease was not the immediate cause of mortality. The 2-year survival rate was 75.8% and the 5-year overall survival rate, 62.1%. The probability of no local and regional tumor disease was 87.7% after 2 years and 81% after 5 years.

Alho and colleagues[37] in a retrospective cohort study recently correlated the prognostic significance of comorbidity for an individual patient with head and neck cancer in regards to age, tumor site, and cancer stage. They concluded that the excess risk associated with comorbidity was confined to subjects less than 65 years old and those with tongue or laryngeal tumors or stage I to II cancer.

Coatesworth[38] conducted a prevalence study of 106 deaths caused by squamous cell cancer of the head and neck. Forty-five deaths (42.5%) were due to locally advanced squamous cell cancer, which represented the larynx, hypopharynx, oropharynx, and oral cavity. Four deaths where due to hemorrhage with locally advanced disease, 19 (18%) to metastatic head and neck cancer, 17 to disseminated malignant disease, and 8 to a second primary (4 lung, 2 esophagus, 1 large bowel, 1 bladder). Pneumonia was the cause of death in 10 cases, and chronic obstructive pulmonary disease in one case. Twenty-three deaths (over 50%) were due to nonmalignant death. The fact that almost one third of the deaths were due to metastatic disease and the suspicion that the eight second primaries were likely unidentified metastases highlight the importance of finding metastases early. Additionally, it is important to note that the majority of deaths were not due to cancer.

SPECIAL TOPICS
Cancer Cachexia

Greater than 50% of patients with advanced head and neck cancer have significant weight loss and possible cachexia.[39] Overall, cachexia accounts for 20% of all cancer-related deaths.[40] It is important to understand the difference between cancer cachexia and starvation, because they are distinctly different entities. In starvation, lean body mass is conserved, and there is a preferential increase in fat metabolism in the liver to supply energy. Ketone bodies from this fat metabolism provide energy for the brain. Additionally, these patients have lower resting energy expenditure, which matches their reduced energy intake. Cancer cachexia appears to be a very different process. It involves the preferential loss of skeletal muscle over adipose tissue, with increased proteolysis and lipolysis, increased metabolic activity of the liver, and increased production of acute phase proteins. In contrast to starvation, cancer cachexia involves inappropriate elevation of resting energy expenditure in many tumor types, even as energy intake may be reduced due to anorexia.[41] Patients with cachexia have generalized asthenia, marked unintentional weight loss, sarcopenia, anemia, anorexia, and emotional and mental fatigue, all of which cause a general decline in functional status. It has been suggested that the treatment of cachexia may improve quality of life.[42]

In a landmark study, Dewys[43] assessed the prognostic effect of weight before chemotherapy. Patients with cachexia-induced weight loss ($\geq 5\%$ body weight lost involuntarily) experienced shorter median survival times than cancer patients without weight loss. Patients with weight loss had poorer responses to chemotherapy and experienced more treatment toxicities. Nguyen and Yueh looked specifically at head and neck squamous cell carcinoma and noted that a weight loss of greater than 10% had a strong prognostic impact on 1-year survival and could be used to predict mortality after recurrent oral cavity and oropharyngeal carcinomas in a retrospective review. They observed that survival was poorest in patients with greater than 10% weight loss at the time of recurrence and best for patients with no weight loss.[44]

Cachexia treatment should incorporate increasing nutritional intake with agents that inhibit muscle and fat wasting and possibly reduce the patient's inflammatory response. Glucocorticosteroids are a commonly used class of agents that have shown short-term improvement in performance status and sense of well-being, as well as increased appetite and food consumption, but not increased body weight.[45] Dexamethasone, which exhibits the least amount of mineralocorticoid activity, has been identified as the steroid of choice in the treatment of cachexia.[46] It may be an appropriate choice for use in patients with limited life expectancy because the side effects may be significant, especially with prolonged use (4–6 weeks), and may include osteoporosis, proximal muscle weakness, immunosuppression, and delirium. Dexamethasone may itself induce skeletal muscle atrophy.[47] Perhaps the most potent appetite stimulant or orexigenic agent is megestrol acetate. Weight gain has been confirmed in some studies of megestrol acetate use in head and neck cancer patients, but it is not clear whether any effect on lean body mass is present.[48] Another alternative is dronabinol (delta-9-tetrahydrocannabinol), a synthetic cannabinoid that has important antiemetic properties. No increase in weight was seen when this agent was administered to patients with advanced cancer, but increased mood and appetite were noted.[49] Current studies with pharmaconutritional support, such as n-3 fatty acids, antioxidant vitamins A and E, and the selective cyclooxygenase (COX-2) inhibitor celecoxib have shown promise.[42]

Legal Issues

Careful planning for the end of life is necessary to ensure that wishes are performed and personal and financial matters are in order. Brain death is recognized as the irreversible end of all brain activity, whereas a persistent vegetative state is when a patient is in a state of coma and has awareness without being wakeful. Some of the most common legal options that persons have during their last days are described herein. As a disclaimer, the reader should consult their state laws, because there are variations and different standards between the states, but this will serve as a general outline.

Advanced directive

An advanced directive is a written legal document that asserts a person's wishes if he or she cannot communicate them any longer. These directives normally cover life-sustaining or heroic measures such as artificial feeding and artificial ventilation. Changes to these documents can be made as long as one is found to still be of sound mind. The two most common forms of an advanced directive are a durable power of attorney and a living will.

Durable power of attorney/health care proxy This legal document names someone who will make all of one's health care decisions if they are unable to. Within it, the person is still able to state his or wishes to be performed. The proxy will have complete control over the decisions made (except for contradicting previously stated wishes) unless one specifically limits their powers.

Living will This document is a statement of a person's wishes to be performed if he or she is unable. It usually involves specific situations that may arise. This form does not appoint a surrogate to make decisions. Because most durable power of attorney documents include these types of instructions, some states do not recognize this as a separate legal document.

End-of-life specific orders

Comfort care only These declarations are a standing set of orders that adhere to the goal of palliative care by directing that efforts to combat the disease process are stopped and the disease be allowed to take its course, with the goal of controlling the unpleasant symptoms that are inevitable, such as pain, nausea, and vomiting.

Do not intubate This order expresses the wish of a patient to forgo mechanical ventilation. Tracheotomy is a form of intubation; therefore, it should be considered carefully.

Do not resuscitate The advent of defibrillation in the 1960s allowed for the reversal of cardiac arrest. Due to the underlying disease process, this intervention is often only temporary, and this order allows a patient to forgo this heroic measure. In addition, the administration of intravenous fluids, blood products, and medications that can affect the heart are considered part of resuscitation.

Hospice care Hospice is a multidisciplinary program designed to increase the quality of life for a person at the end of life but does not require that the patient be in a do not resuscitate status. This program can be administered where the patient chooses, that is, a nursing home, the home of a relative, or in their own home. Types of support offered may include medical, emotional, spiritual, and therapy. Often, a component is offered for the family of the patient, which can include counseling, bereavement help, support groups, and training in how to care for their loved one.

Medical marijuana

Medical marijuana has been touted by its proponents for benefits in palliative care such as antiemetic properties and appetite stimulation, but its status as a prohibited drug makes its use controversial and most times illegal. Since 1996, 12 states have legalized medical marijuana use: Arkansas, California, Colorado, Hawaii, Maine,

Montana, Nevada, New Mexico, Oregon, Rhode Island, Vermont, and Washington.[50] Cannabinoids, along with palliative benefits in cancer therapy, have been associated with anticarcinogenic effects. The antiproliferative activities of cannabinoids have been intensively investigated.[51,52] Ramer and Hinz[53] set out to study the effects of cannabinoids on tumor invasion. They discovered that methanandamide and tetrahydrocannabinol (THC) caused a time- and concentration-dependent suppression of human cervical cancer cell invasion, which was accompanied by increased expression of tissue inhibitors of matrix metalloproteinases (TIMP), specifically TIMP-1.

A study by Naef and colleagues[54] compared the effects of THC, morphine, morphine plus THC, and placebo in an effort to learn about each combination's effect on different types of pain. They artificially created pain scenerios of cold, heat, pressure, and electrical stimulation. Overall they found that THC did not significantly reduce pain. In the cold and heat tests, it even produced hyperalgesia, which was completely neutralized by THC plus morphine. A slight additive analgesic effect was observed for THC plus morphine in the electrical stimulation test. No analgesic effect resulted in the pressure and heat test with THC or THC plus morphine.

SUMMARY

Palliative care in patients who have head and neck cancer is a complex topic that requires a multifaceted approach. It is imperative for the surgeon to discuss incurable cancer with the patient and family openly and honestly. Communication is the key to success. A multifaceted team including a cancer nurse, nurse practitioner, and cancer patient navigator is important. The patient should be encouraged to deal with legal issues including code status and advance directives. This preparation allays anxiety for the family and health care provider in the event of a catastrophic emergency. The surgical team should be aware of patient and family support groups and hospice care in their area of residence. The principle of maintenance of quality of life should be held supreme, and the options given to patients should encompass nonsurgical and surgical therapies. Xerostomia, although seemingly an inconsequential side effect of radiation, uniformly worsens the quality of life of cancer patients. The head and neck surgeon has an important duty to fulfill in managing and following the wishes of the incurable cancer patient and is obligated to direct them to the appropriate services in this challenging time.

REFERENCES

1. Ellershaw, Ward C. Care of the dying patient: the last hours or days of life. BMJ 2003;326:30–4.
2. Cohen LM, Poppel DM, Cohn GM, et al. A very good death: measuring quality of dying in end stage renal disease. J Palliat Med 2001;4:167–72.
3. Fried T, van Droom C, O'Leary J, et al. Older persons' preference for site of terminal care. Ann Intern Med 1999;131:109–12.
4. Steinhauser KE, Clipp EC, McNeilly CM, et al. In search of a good death: observations of patients, families and providers. Ann Intern Med 2000;132:825–32.
5. van den Beuken-van Everdingen MH, de Rijke JM, Kessels AG, et al. Prevalence of pain in patients with cancer: a systematic review of the past 40 years. Ann Oncol 2007;18(9):1437–49.
6. Kowalski LP, Carvalho AL. Natural history of untreated head and neck cancer. Eur J Cancer 2000;36:1032–7.
7. Hallenbeck JL, Stratos GA, Katz S. Stanford faculty development program in end-of-life care. Stanford, CA: Stanford University School of Medicine; 2000.

8. Graf R, Hildebrandt B, Tilly W, et al. A non-randomized, single-centre comparison of induction chemotherapy followed by radiochemotherapy versus concomitant chemotherapy with hyperfractionated radiotherapy in inoperable head and neck carcinomas. BMC Cancer 2006;6(30):1–9.
9. Yogi V, Singh OP. Induction followed with concurrent chemoradiotherapy in advanced head and neck cancer. J Cancer Res Ther 2005;1(4):198–203.
10. Mohanti BK, Umapathy H, Bahadur S, et al. Short course palliative radiotherapy of 20 Gy in 5 fractions for advanced and incurable head and neck cancer: AIIMS study. Radiother Oncol 2004;71(3):275–80.
11. Teymoortash A, Bien S, Dalchow C, et al. Selective high-dose intra-arterial cis-platin as palliative treatment for incurable head and neck cancer. Onkologie 2004;27(6):547–51.
12. Forbes JF. Palliative surgery in cancer patients: principles and potential of palliative surgery in patients with advanced cancer. Recent Results Cancer Res 1988; 108:134–42.
13. Lim RY. Laser tumor debulking. West Virginia Medical Journal 1989;85(12):530–2.
14. Laccourreye O, Lawson G, Muscatello L, et al. Carbon dioxide laser debulking for obstructing endolaryngeal carcinoma: a 10-year experience. Ann Otol Rhinol Laryngol 1999;108(5):490–4.
15. Phelan E, Lang E, Mahesh BN, et al. Powered instrumentation in obstructing laryngeal tumours. J Laryngol Otol 2007;121(3):293–5.
16. Paleri V, Stafford FW, Sammut MS. Laser debulking in malignant upper airway obstruction. Head Neck 2005;27(4):296–301.
17. Halfpenny W, McGurk M. Stomal recurrence following temporary tracheostomy. J Laryngol Otol 2001;115:202–4.
18. Grocott P. The palliative management of fungating malignant wounds. J Wound Care 2000;9(1):4–9.
19. Morrison M. A colour guide to the nursing management of wounds. London: Wolfe; 1992.
20. Rumsey N, Clarke A, White P. Exploring the psychosocial concerns of outpatients with disfiguring conditions. J Wound Care 2003;12(7):247–52.
21. Katz MR, Irish JC, Devins GM, et al. Communicating in the patient without a larynx. Head Neck 2002;25(2):103–12.
22. Sandel HD, Davison SP. Microsurgical reconstruction for radiation necrosis: an evolving disease. J Reconstr Microsurg 2007;23:225–30.
23. Volpato LE, Silva TC, Oliveira TM, et al. Radiation therapy and chemotherapy-induced oral mucositis. Rev Bras Otorrinolaringol 2007;73(4):562–8.
24. Elting LS, Cooksley CD, Chambers MS, et al. Risk, outcomes, and costs of radiation-induced oral mucositis among patients with head-and-neck malignancies. Int J Radiat Oncol Biol Phys 2007;68:1110–20.
25. Aziz L, Ebenfelt A. Mucosal secretion changes during radiotherapy in the oral cavity. Clin Oral Investig 2007;11(3):293–6.
26. Patni N, Patni S, Bapna A. The optimal use of granulocyte macrophage colony stimulating factor in radiation induced mucositis in head and neck squamous cell carcinoma. J Cancer Res Ther 2005;1(3):136–41.
27. Veerasarn V, Phromratanapongse P, Suntornpong N, et al. Effect of amifostine to prevent radiotherapy-induced acute and late toxicity in head and neck cancer patients who had normal or mild impaired salivary gland function. J Med Assoc Thai 2006;89(12):2056–67.
28. Penpattanagul S. Reduced incidence and severity of acute radiation mucositis by WF10 (IMMUNOKINE) as adjunct to standard of care in the

management of head and neck cancer patients. J Med Assoc Thai 2007; 90(8):1590–600.

29. Rydholm M, Strang P. Physical and psychosocial impact of xerostomia in palliative cancer care: a qualitative interview study. Int J Palliat Nurs 2002;8(7):318–23.

30. Jellema AP, Slotman BJ, Doornaert P, et al. Impact of radiation-induced xerostomia on quality of life after primary radiotherapy among patients with head and neck cancer. Int J Radiat Oncol Biol Phys 2007;69(3):751–60.

31. Davies AN, Brailsford SR, Beighton D. Oral candidosis in patients with advanced cancer. Oral Oncol 2006;42(7):698–702.

32. Feio M, Sapeta P. Xerostomia in palliative care. Acta Med Port 2005;18(6):459–65.

33. Hargitai IA, Sherman RG, Strother JM. The effects of electrostimulation on parotid saliva flow: a pilot study. Oral Surg Oral Med Oral Pathol Oral Radiol Endod 2005;99(3):316–20.

34. Takakura K, Takaki S, Takeda I, et al. Effect of cevimeline on radiation-induced salivary gland dysfunction and AQP5 in submandibular gland in mice. Bull Tokyo Dent Coll 2007;48(2):47–56.

35. Kahn ST, Johnstone PA. Management of xerostomia related to radiotherapy for head and neck cancer. Oncology (Williston Park) 2005;19(14):1827–32 [discussion: 1832–4, 1837–9].

36. Wutzl A, Ploder O, Kermer C, et al. Mortality and causes of death after multimodality treatment for advanced oral and oropharyngeal cancer. J Oral Maxillofac Surg 2007;65(2):255–60.

37. Alho OP, Hannula K, Luokkala A, et al. Differential prognostic impact of comorbidity in head and neck cancer. Head Neck 2007;29(10):913–8.

38. Coatesworth AP, Tsikoudas A, MacLennan K. The cause of death in patients with head and neck squamous cell carcinoma. J Laryngol Otol 2002;116:269–71.

39. Lees J. Incidence of weight loss in head and neck cancer patients on commencing radiotherapy treatment at a regional oncology center. Eur J Cancer Care 1999;8:133–6.

40. Inagaki J, Rodriquez V, Bodey GP. Causes of death in cancer patients. Cancer 1974;33:568–71.

41. Tisdale MJ. Cachexia in cancer patients. Nature 2002;2:862–71.

42. Mantovani G, Mededdu C, Maccio A, et al. Cancer-related anorexia/cachexia syndrome and oxidative stress: an innovative approach beyond current treatment. Cancer Epidermiol Biomarkers Prev 2004;13:1651–9.

43. Dewys WD. Weight loss and nutritional abnormalities in cancer patients: incidence, severity and significance. Clin Oncol 1986;5:251.

44. Nguyen TV, Yueh B. Weight loss predicts morality after recurrent oral cavity and oropharyngeal carcinomas. Cancer 2002;52:72–91.

45. Inui A. Cancer anorexia-cachexia syndrome: current issues in research and management. CA Cancer J Clin 2002;52:72–91.

46. Von Roenn JH, Paice JA. Control of common, non-pain cancer symptoms. Semin Oncol 2005;32:200–10.

47. Stitt TN, Drujan D, Clarke BA, et al. The IGF-1/PI3K/Akt pathway prevents expression of muscle atrophy-induced ubiquitin ligases by inhibiting FOXO transcription factors. Mol Cell 2004;14:395–403.

48. Mantovani G, Maccio A, Bianchi A, et al. Megestrol acetate in neoplastic anorexia/cachexia: clinical evaluation and comparison with cytokine levels in patients with head and neck carcinoma treated with neoadjuvant chemotherapy. Int J Clin Lab Res 1995;25:135–41.

49. Nelson K, Walsh D, Deeter P, et al. A phase II study of delta-9-tetrahydrocannabinol for appetite stimulation in cancer-associated anorexia. J Palliat Care 1994;10: 14–8.

50. Drug War Facts. States with legalized medical marijuana. Available at: http://www.drugwarfacts.org/medicalm.htm. Accessed May 20, 2008.
51. Massi P, Valenti M, Vaccani A, et al. 5-Lipoxygenase and anandamide hydrolase (FAAH) mediate the antitumor activity of cannabidiol, a non-psychoactive cannabinoid. J Neurochem 2008;104(4):1091–100.
52. Parolaro D, Massi P. Cannabinoids as potential new therapy for the treatment of gliomas. Expert Rev Neurother 2008;8(1):37–49.
53. Ramer R, Hinz B. Inhibition of cancer cell invasion by cannabinoids via increased expression of tissue inhibitor of matrix metalloproteinases-1. J Natl Cancer Inst 2008;100(1):59–69.
54. Naef M, Curatolo M, Petersen-Felix S, et al. The analgesic effect of oral delta-9-tetrahydrocannabinol (THC), morphine, and a THC-morphine combination in healthy subjects under experimental pain conditions. Pain 2003;105(1–2):79–88.

Index

Note: Page numbers of article titles are in **boldface** type.

A

Affect component-affective disorders, in tinnitus, 30
Airway endoscopy, in recurrent respiratory papillomatosis, 59–60
Alzheimer's disease, olfactory deficits in, 127–128
Amyotrophic lateral sclerosis, dysphagia in, 90
    speech problems in, 108–109
    tracheostomy in, 139–140
Anosmia, in elderly, **123–131**
Antibiotic therapy, in refractory chronic rhinosinusitis, 43, 44
Antifungal therapy, in refractory chronic rhinosinusitis, 45
Antiviral therapy, in recurrent respiratory papillomatosis, 63–64
Anxiety, chronic subjective dizziness with, 73–74

B

Balance disorder patient, exercises for, progression of, 164
    vestibular exercise for, 165
    vestibular rehabilitation in, **161–169**
        adaptation in, 162–163
        efficacy of, 166–167
        habitation in, 162
        in recovery of function, 166–167
        substitution in, 163–165

C

Cachexia, due to cancer of head and neck, 178–179
Cancer, of head and neck. See *Head and neck, cancer of.*
Cerebrovascular accident, dysphonia in, 111
Cerebrovascular disease, dysphagia in, 92–93
Cerebrovascular factors, in tinnitus, 29
Cervical articular blocks, 156, 157
Cervical medial blocks, 157
Chemoradiation therapy, in cancer of head and neck, 171–172
Cochlear implants, in sensorineural hearing loss, 83–84
Cognitive-based therapy, in tinnitus, 31–32
Cranial base surgery, evaluation for, 49–50
    palatal adhesion technique and, 54, 55
    rehabilitation after, **49–56**
    vocal fold medialization technique and, 55–56
Cranial nerve deficits, cranial base surgery in, 50–54
Cricoid resection, in dysphagia, 95

Otolaryngol Clin N Am 42 (2009) 185–191
doi:10.1016/S0030-6665(08)00185-0
0030-6665/08/$ – see front matter © 2009 Elsevier Inc. All rights reserved.

Moving?

Make sure your subscription moves with you!

To notify us of your new address, find your **Clinics Account Number** (located on your mailing label above your name), and contact customer service at:

E-mail: elspcs@elsevier.com

800-654-2452 (subscribers in the U.S. & Canada)
314-453-7041 (subscribers outside of the U.S. & Canada)

Fax number: 314-523-5170

Elsevier Periodicals Customer Service
11830 Westline Industrial Drive
St. Louis, MO 63146

*To ensure uninterrupted delivery of your subscription, please notify us at least 4 weeks in advance of move.

Printed and bound by CPI Group (UK) Ltd, Croydon, CR0 4YY

03/10/2024

01040443-0020